MW01245387

The HEART *of* HEALTH

Avoiding Deception

JAMES L. MARCUM, M.D.
with Charles Mills

Unless otherwise noted, texts are from the Holy Bible, New International Version. Copyright © 1973, 1978, 1984, International Bible Society. Used by permission of Zondervan Bible Publishers.

Texts credited to NKJV are from the New King James Version. Copyright © 1979, 1980, 1983 by Thomas Nelson, Inc. Used by permission. All rights reserved.

Book editor: Charles Mills
Copy editor: Delma Miller
Cover designer: Ron Pride
Layout: Tami Pohle

Library of Congress Control Number: 2010913332
ISBN: 978-0-578-05968-6
Copyright © 2010 by James L. Marcum II, M.D.
Ooltewah, Tennessee 37363
All Rights Reserved
Printed in the United States of America

Disclaimer: The information in this book is not intended to be a substitute for expert medical advice or treatment. Every individual has unique characteristics. This book should not supersede the advice of your physicians.

Dedication

I would like to dedicate this book to my parents, Jim and Mary Marcum,
who have taught and supported me throughout my life.
They have focused my learning on what the Great Physician teaches.
This book exists because of their love and guidance.
Dr. James Marcum

To Dorinda, who brings health and healing into my life every day.
Charles Mills

Acknowledgments

There are many who have contributed to this project. I hope they realize how important they are to me. Charles Mills is more than a "with." He has been a friend, mentor, and a gigantic creative force. Through his years of work and experience, he has brought together the ideas given to me by the Holy Spirit and merged them with the insights shared by the many healers he has interviewed and admired through the years.

I would also like to express thanks to Dorinda Mills, who I know is always there supporting and contributing to Charles' ministry.

A thumbs-up to Ron Pride, who designed the cover; Delma Miller, who carefully copyedited each word; designer Tami Pohle for creating a very readable layout; Brad Fisher at College Press; Neal Ardmon, Lou Seals, Henry Luken and my friends at Retro, who have all played vital roles in the production process.

I could not have completed this project without the support of my loving wife, Sonya, and children Kelli and Jake. You are the best.

A special note of appreciation to my office staff at the Chattanooga Heart Institute, Arvid and Doreen Jacobson, Steve Gallimore and staff at LifeTalk, and my many patients and friends who have helped this project become a reality. You blessed my life and have been a part of the 20-year journey of this book.

Finally, I want to say a special thanks and praise to my God who has guided this book all along through the Holy Spirit. To Him all glory be given. His love and patience are always appreciated.

Contents

Introduction

You and I are, at this moment, part of the largest, most comprehensive health study this world has ever known. It's not being funded by any well-respected organization like the National Institutes of Health or the American Medical Association. There are no highly trained scientists bending low over colorful test tubes or peering pensively into glowing microscopes searching for subtle clues. No forms are being completed or random samples taken. This study is quietly, unobtrusively being carried out in our homes, our schools, and in our places of business.

The goal of this incredible, far-reaching investigation is to answer three very simple questions. The first is, What happens to the human body when it does everything . . . wrong? What happens when it's continually fed toxic, nutritionally deficient foods, robbed of necessary sleep, deprived of vital water intake, inundated with a steady stream of harsh chemicals, introduced to a never-ending supply of devastating, side-effect-laden pharmaceuticals, and is forced to breathe in a constant flow of polluted air?

The second question is similar to the first, but has to do with the human mind: What happens when the information pouring into a brain's neural network is wrong; when it's taught to focus entirely on its own needs, its own desires, and its own happiness at the expense of all else?

And finally, the study is examining our spiritual lives, asking the question: What happens to a person's relationship with God when that relationship is based on beliefs that are built on flawed foundations; on images of God that are totally, heartbreakingly wrong?

The results are pouring in. You can see them at the mall, on television, the Internet, and standing in line at the bank. You can catch glimpses of them as you talk with coworkers or even strangers on the street, when you read the blogs of "experts" on the Web, and when you scan your evening news source. You can see them at your local church, in the halls of Congress, and especially in crowded doctors' offices.

Many of us see the results of that ongoing study reflected back to us from our own mirrors. We stand gazing into the face of an overweight, overworked, overstimulated person we hardly recognize. We lean forward and squint into the eyes of someone who hasn't a clue about what's going on inside his or her own body, yet we know all isn't right in there—something very bad is happening deep inside us. We understand, although we don't know how or why, something important is missing—something necessary for the days, weeks, and years ahead. But, all we can do is stand there, unsure, confused, and afraid.

That's what happens when the human body, mind, and spirit become so wrapped up with what tastes good, feels good, and seems good that we lose sight of what *is* good. That's what happens when truth is hidden, and questioning people start to depend on a random set of highly polished, expertly marketed, and decidedly deadly . . . lies.

In the condition civilization has placed itself, doctors often don't know what to do beyond treating symptoms and hoping for the best. Psychiatrists shake their heads in disbelief, wondering how their patients could ever get so emotionally messed up when they have so much for which to live. Pastors gaze down from their pulpits at dwindling flocks, searching for a way to transform what has become an unattractive, seemingly inattentive, and reportedly highly agitated God into something worth worshipping. And parents stand helplessly by watching as their children are attacked by diseases that used to inflict only the elderly, all the while trying to juggle their overstretched budget to cover astronomical medical insurance costs and the growing list of prescription drugs.

Very Different

It hasn't always been this way. One hundred years ago, the world was a very different place filled with people living a very different life. Most families grew and ate their own food. We didn't process our nourishment with heavy amounts of fats, salt, and added calories. Obesity, diabetes, heart disease, and many forms of cancers were rare. Social life was centered around the family unit and the local church was the hub of activity in a town. A majority enjoyed a weekly day of rest and the Bible was the most-read book in the home. Physical activity? That went hand in hand with what it took to survive or simply put food on the table. We walked places instead of riding, drank water instead of soda, went to bed with the sun instead of after the late news, and found pleasure in creative—not passive—outlets.

The only health-care crisis existing was whether Doc Brown could get through the snowstorm in time to treat a broken limb or help deliver a baby.

The world has changed. Today, we eat out of convenience, dumping copious amounts of highly processed foods down our throats, hardly ever glancing at nutrition labels. Our cuisine is saturated with chemicals placed there to preserve "freshness" and turn us into addicts who will keep coming back for more. Television commercials scream their audio-enhanced messages urging overconsumption as families eat on the run, rarely sitting down to enjoy a meal together.

We listen to iPhones instead of birds chirping. We spend more time indoors than out. We let the media define our thoughts, telling us what's important in life. Texting is replacing talking. Watching is replacing reading. Like sheep without a shepherd, we're allowing "media darlings" and other random strangers to dictate our thoughts and agendas. We're overmedicated and undernourished. The family unit is eroding and God is becoming less and less important in our lives. When we finally exhaust ourselves in our constant strain for everything, all the time, some look around at their lives, judge them worthless, and commit suicide in increasing numbers. The rest of us simply stare into our mirrors wondering why we're so sick all the time.

I have some good news for you, and you don't have to be a rocket scientist to understand it. We're in this tragic condition because we were not designed to live this life. It's as simple as that. The One who made us, who lovingly formed us from the "dust of the ground" according to Genesis 2:7, had a very different lifestyle in mind. We were designed to live in harmony with nature, not manipulate it to our liking or financial gain. We were created to live a life free of undue stress, not run ourselves 24/7 as though less was unacceptable. We were supposed to be creative creatures, not passive couch potatoes spending our lives being entertained by the creative efforts of others. Most important of all, we were designed to worship the God who made us, not spend our lives running away from Him.

In short, we were designed to love each other, care for the earth, and worship our Creator. The further we distance ourselves from that ideal, the sicker we become.

Where Do I Start?

When I sat down to write this book, I was almost overwhelmed by the challenges ahead. Where should I start? What should be the very first words? How could I bring to the world a plan of action that would make a real difference in lives; that would change people; that could literally save them from years of disease and suffering? Should I use a scientific approach and find double-blinded, randomized, placebo-controlled trials to prove and promote the truths found in the original human "Owner's Manual," the Bible? The scientific community would certainly appreciate that approach. Should I compile all the great works of God's healers throughout time and weave them into one gigantic volume? The literary community would be thrilled.

But in the quiet of soul-searching contemplation, I felt God asking me to write about the things I have seen and heard over the years I have practiced medicine as a cardiologist. I want this book to be personal—me talking to you about what I've discovered in my continuing journey to be at the very heart of health. I want to share with you, not only as doctor-to-patient but as friend-to-friend, the many deceptions clouding our lives and making us sick.

Am I qualified to do this? Why should you want to read a book by James Marcum? What makes him so special? The answer lies not in the messenger, but in the message. The power of this book is not found in the words and studies and nutritional information you'll read. It's not dependent on the depth of research or degrees held by those quoted. The power of this book is entirely dependent on the work of the Holy Spirit, both in its writing and in its reading.

You see, I "practice" the healing arts. But, God *created* them. And it is to God that I want to refer you, and every patient who comes to see me. Why? Because He is what's missing in this world. He holds the ultimate answer to every illness, every condition, and every heartbreak. He is the Great Physician, the only true healer, the one who can touch lives and make people whole again.

This is why I'm writing this book. Because I believe God has given me a message to share with you.

In the following pages, I plan to introduce you to some of my patients and how the very questions you're asking about your health are being answered in their lives.

Most Influential

I was reading a recent poll of men who were asked who they thought was the most influential male in the world today. This would be the individual whom they looked up to for answers; someone they wanted to emulate.

Number one on the list was Don Draper, a character on a television series. He is not even a real person!

Number two was Usain Bolt, an Olympic athlete who, many believe, defines the true spirit of competition.

President Barack Obama slipped in as number three.

While this poll may or may not reflect the feelings of most men, it was just another example of how the media has the power to create an influential character, market him as an ideal to the world, and affect the minds of a large segment of the population. That same media is doing the same thing when it comes to telling us how to build and maintain optimal health. They are often busily promoting dangerous medications, toxic foods, destructive lifestyles, and dubious cures. Which leads us to the next question, Who controls the media? Who, or *what*, is pulling the strings on the most powerful influence in our world today?

As for the poll, wouldn't it be nice if the most influential man in this world were the man who loves us the most; who provides true answers to life's troubling questions; who is, right at this moment, hovering beside you as you read this book? Wouldn't it be nice if the one who received the most votes the One who longs to hold you in His arms, remembers the day you were born, appreciates the good in you and wants to help eradicate the bad, while building a future for you far exceeding your wildest dreams? Why didn't He make the Top Ten list?

There's a reason. It's because the deceptions under which we are all living include, not only what God does, but what He *is*.

I want you to know the answers you're looking for when it comes to physical, mental, and spiritual healing that can be found in Him.

Are you ready to uncover these deceptions? Are you ready to find the truth in an error-filled world? Then let's begin our journey back to the heart of health.

Chapter 1

Victim of Deception

It was two o'clock on a Wednesday morning when my pager sounded. Tuesday is a "call night" for me, which means I'm available for any and all situations needing my attention at the hospital. I had been on the phone an hour before helping to resolve a minor crisis and was just drifting off to sleep, hoping for a few moments of peace and quiet. I should have known better.

The familiar number illuminated on my pager identified the source. I dialed it quickly and the emergency room doctor picked up on the first ring. "We've got a 38-year-old male experiencing severe chest pain. I'm thinking heart attack."

My colleague was right. The symptoms were common for heart attack or myocardial infarction. I knew the patient in the emergency room was quickly running out of time and if something wasn't done soon, he could die.

When I arrived in the examination room, "the patient" became David. He was now very real to me—a man with pale skin and terrified eyes. I had seen that look before. His blood pressure was dangerously low. He had already received a dose of aspirin and heparin to thin his blood, and was hooked up to oxygen and a continuous heart monitor.

I introduced myself and examined his chart. This was serious, very serious. After saying a quick prayer on my patient's behalf, I began to explain to him that he urgently needed a procedure to open up the artery supplying the front of his heart with blood. A team was being put together to fly him by helicopter to a facility where this operation could take place.

What happened next took only a few moments, but seemed to last forever. These events are frozen in my mind. David slumped down onto the examination table, his face turning white as his heart rhythm became completely random, erratic, and unstable. This rhythm caused the blood in his body to stop circulating—a condition called ventricular tachycardia, then ventricular fibrillation. Within seconds, he passed out completely.

A team of highly skilled caregivers rushed into the room. The shirt on David's chest was removed, and two electrode pads attached to a defibrillator by wires were placed on his bare chest. A shock of electricity jolted his body, causing it to convulse slightly as all eyes turned in hope to the EKG monitor. Sure enough, the wave of lines indicating the patient's heartbeats ceased their wild and random dance and settled once again into a steady *beat, beat, beat.* David's eyes fluttered open and he stared blankly up at me for a moment, unsure of what was going on. "How do you feel?" I asked.

"I'm OK," he responded weakly, glancing about at the other faces in the room, wondering where all these people had come from.

When I asked him about his chest pain, he said it was gone. I noticed his blood pressure and heart rhythm had also normalized. For the moment at least, my patient was out of danger. In reality, David was dying and would have died. He had been pulled back to life using a now common technology. I whispered a prayer of thanks to the God who allows medical professionals to perform "miracles" using the tools found in most modern hospitals.

As preparations for his flight to the operating facility continued, I walked into the waiting room to talk with David's wife, Debbie, and their two teenage daughters. They'd heard the alarms and commotion. They'd seen the technicians running down the hallway. They knew something was very wrong with their husband and daddy. They were terrified. Panic shone in their eyes as they desperately clung to one another trying to maintain sanity.

"How could this happen?" David's wife wanted to know after I explained the situation. "He's never been sick a day in his life!"

How could this happen? It's a question I hear often, and the answer isn't always easy. I told Debbie that I'd explain everything as best I could later. But for now, we had to make sure David was getting the acute care he needed.

David's left anterior descending coronary artery had a 98 percent blockage. His heart simply wasn't receiving enough blood to function optimally. It would be as though your oxygen supply was 98 percent blocked and then you tried to climb a mountain. This situation would affect not only your ability to breathe, but also the ability of every organ in your body to function—including your heart. Blood—pumped by the heart—carries oxygen up to the top of your head and down to the tips of your toes. In essence, when your heart stops functioning correctly, your entire body begins to suffocate. In David's case, this caused chest pain, low blood pressure, and a dangerous heart rhythm.

Within an hour, a stent—a device to keep an artery open—was placed in David's coronary artery so blood could flow freely again. My patient was fortunate that no permanent damage had taken place to his heart or other organs during his sudden heart attack and subsequent cardiac arrest on the examination table. I guess the best place to have a cardiac event is in a hospital while carrying on a conversation with a cardiologist!

This is where some well-meaning people might miss an important point. We hear quite a bit about alternative medicines, potent herbal cures, or the importance of diet and exercise. And I will be the first to champion anything proven to work. But there is, and always will be, a place for modern medicine, *especially* in emergency situations. If I'm having a heart attack, I want a stent. If my heart is going too slow, give me a pacemaker. If I'm bleeding to death, stop the bleeding and start a transfusion. If I have a bacterial infection, bring me some antibiotics. Without modern medicine, many people would not be around to explore alternative medicines, examine herbal cures, or learn the importance of diet and exercise.

David was suffering an acute event brought on by a chronic condition. As I later dug into his history, I began to understand why he ended up on my examination table. His heart disease was caused by elements in his life bringing stress on his body. He smoked. He held a high-pressure job. He ate food practically devoid of nutrition. But did he, his wife, or his two precious daughters recognize those stressors as the cause of his heart disease? No. Why? Because they, like many of us, are being deceived. No one is making the connection for them.

First Deception

What is a deception anyway? Doesn't it depend on a point of view or perception? Not really. A deception is a falsehood, a lie, a trick, an untruth. Deceptions are all around us and have been going on since the beginning of time. Sometimes the deceptions are so elaborate even the most astute don't recognize the untruth. Ninety-eight percent truth is still a deception. Good people—intelligent people—are being deceived or have become clueless concerning certain facts of life. Why? Amazingly, it usually—as we'll discover—comes down to money.

More specifically, I want to suggest that deception exists because of selfishness. We—and the society in which we live—put our own interests above the interests of others. This often centers on money, power, and control.

One current deception is the thought that modern medicine can fix anything. To be brutally honest, modern medicine usually does not fix anything. But it does a pretty good job of dealing with the symptoms of a lot of things.

"Oh, but Doctor Marcum," I hear you say. "How about a broken leg? Doesn't a doctor fix that?"

The doctor can *set* the leg. He can make it so you don't have to limp for the rest of your life. But as for the healing of the broken bone, the doctor can only watch and be amazed.

"How about cancer? Don't we praise God for cancer survivors?"

Absolutely! But many who receive the same treatment, experience the same therapy, go through the same procedures, succumb to their disease. Regardless of the survival rate, often disease is not fixed. At best, we'd have to say the rampaging cancer was slowed—which is a good thing indeed. Life was extended by modern medicine. Unfortunately, the extension often comes with a price, including side effects and collateral damage to other organs.

Here's the scary part. People who experience heart disease, who suffer from cancer, who fight debilitating pains, who stand in lines at drugstores waiting to fill their endless prescriptions, who sit and watch television commercials extolling the power of the latest and greatest pharmaceutical, firmly believe their doctors or the pills given are providing a cure to their ills. They think they're getting "fixed." They are usually wrong.

So what do we do when we are facing a health crisis? The short answer is: "Depends on the crisis." The longer answer is: "Depends on the cause of the crisis."

I divide illness into two categories: acute illness and chronic illness. "Acute" means "something needs to be done right now, this second, or you might die." That certainly describes my patient David as his heart malfunctioned on the examination table. He needed action—and he needed it now.

"Chronic" means "ongoing, frequent duration, always present." While David's heart attack was sudden and acute, it was the result of something going on for a very long time. Arteries don't just fill up with plaque overnight. That is why when his wife asked, "How could this happen?" I knew I needed more information about my patient before I could answer completely. His heart attack wasn't the problem. It was the *result* of the problem.

Modern medical technology can be breathtaking in its effectiveness to treat acute illnesses. Most people are completely unaware of what goes on behind the closed doors of science laboratories and medical institutions. Our ability to learn and understand the universe and the human body is expanding faster than at any time in history. Force fields are no longer science fiction. Machines can now render objects invisible. Using atom smashers, scientists are hoping to discover more about the universe and the relationships between energy and matter. With enough energy, scientists are hoping to *create* matter. Teleportation of matter is more than a theory at this point. Many discoveries are being kept secret because of their military significance.

There are now computers performing unbelievable computations. Our DNA has been sequenced—providing a glimpse into the past, present, and future. I have been reading about something called nanotechnology by which scientists are making very, very small particles capable of penetrating into cells, diagnosing a problem, and delivering specialized treatments to address the problem.

Yes, there is a place for technology. But this expansion of knowledge is accomplishing something unexpected. Using technology, we are also now able to measure and quantitate situations such as worship and how this act can change chemical reactions in our bodies—reactions affecting every cell, muscle, and organ. We can identify and show how rest, nutrition, and even laughter help cure our ills and strengthen our immune system. Seems we have many other newly developing treatments to fight disease at the cellular level. All too often many are not being told this. And there's a reason, which we'll identify later.

But there is a downside to advancing technology. As technology expands, we tend to look more and more at what *we* can do as human beings. We start worshipping at the altar of science instead of at the feet of the One who made us. As we start to see our symptoms diminish, we think we've found a cure. Who needs God? And the deception deepens.

The most important question we need to be asking ourselves is not "How can we get well?" but rather, "Why are we sick?" This is the question that can lead to finding the "ultimate fix."

Number One Killer

Cardiovascular disease is the number one killer in America, and its worldwide prevalence continues to rise. Some sources say doctors, hospitals, medications, overdoseages, and medical errors are surpassing cardiovascular disease as the number one source of death, and this may be true and is certainly a shame. But both statistics support the same conclusion. Neither patient nor doctor is clear on what causes many of our health problems or how best to combat them. We must strive to understand the cause and not merely be satisfied with treating symptoms.

Presently, one common theory blames inflammation. Another theory is the real cause of cardiovascular disease is genetic. But genetic alterations take many, many generations to develop. Heart disease was practically unheard of a hundred years ago and there are still places on earth where very few suffer from this condition.

In about half the cases of cardiovascular disease, the first manifestation is a heart attack. In other words, the patient does not know heart disease is a problem under construction. The first symptom is like David's—a heart attack. Education is crucial. Reading this book may save your life or the life of a loved one.

Over the next 24 hours, around 3,000 American hearts will malfunction. This is nearly the same number of persons who died in the tragedy of September 11, 2001. This comes to 1.1 million heart attacks a year. One out of three will die at the time of the initial event or within the first 12 months after.

Forty percent of Americans have cardiovascular disease of some sort, and in women the death rate from this condition is eight times higher than the death rate from cancer. In fact, in women, cardiovascular disease poses a greater risk than breast cancer and all other diseases *combined*. Those numbers continue to climb.

I am now going to say something that may startle and even anger you. But I'm just the messenger, so please hold your wrath in check. Some estimate that 90 percent of cardiovascular disease is acquired. That's right. The painful truth is we give the disease to ourselves by the choices we make during a lifetime. We create the chronic condition bringing about the acute event by placing endless stressors on our systems—stressors that may, eventually, end our lives.

In David's case, he didn't even know he had a problem until that early

Wednesday morning when it felt like an elephant sat down to rest on his chest. I thank God that after this experience he began his search for what was at the heart of his problem—at the heart of health. When he was faced with death, he started to evaluate the reason he had a heart attack.

Chapter 2

Searching for Truth

There are many health professionals (and pseudoprofessionals) currently promoting everything from live-longer potions and build-your-immune-system supplements to super healthy eating plans and counteracting-dangerous-toxins creams. We see them on infomercials, hear them on talk radio, click on their interactive Web sites, and read their colorful books. Some make a lot of sense. Some make no sense at all.

A few stress balance, but most harp on their own area of interest or financial gain as if nothing else matters. They drive home their message wrapped in a polished and convincing sales pitch. Some are sincere. Others only want to make a buck. Some give good information. Others present partial truths. All proclaim they have found the answer to your "unique" health problem. They say they have found *the* answer. If only it were that simple.

How do we put this clamor of information together to make sense? How does an average person who lives an average life know what to believe, whom to believe, or what the next step should be in achieving a healthy life? Do we wait for a governmental regulation or the family physician to tell us what to do? Do we take personal responsibility? Do the answers really exist?

Take high fructose corn syrup for example. We hear that it's killing us. Surely our government would not allow it on the market and our local hospitals would not be serving it to patients if this were true. We hear when we eat this ingredient, our body doesn't make leptin as it should. Leptin is a chemical that makes us feel full and satisfied. Therefore, without leptin we eat more than we should and become fat. Yet, high fructose corn syrup is listed among the ingredients of many of our favorite foods and is neatly tucked inside many of the selections on the hospital menu.

We know argon is a chemical put on fruits and vegetables making them look great and possibly harming us in the process. Yet, the fruits and vegetables we find in many grocery stores are coated with argon. What's going on?

While I cannot address every harmful food, dangerous toxin, dubious treatment, or hidden deception out there, I can give you a framework and approach to use as you face these apparent contradictions. This is the approach I began to take with David in his search for the reason he had a heart attack.

The first thing you should understand is that by discovering what the body needs, we can often uncover much about what the body does *not* need. For instance, most of our body is comprised of water. It's essential for chemical reactions. Our bodies not only need but actually, at times, crave water. It's the most important substance needed for our machine to run efficiently and properly. We know this because without a steady and sufficient supply of water we would soon die. So we can safely conclude that foods with low water content may not be what is best for us. True, our bodies can extract water from whatever food we eat, but here is an interesting fact. While most Americans are overweight, we are also severely dehydrated. This indicates that what most Americans eat—and drink—does not contain the water they need. So, if you're thirsty, you can just know your body is not asking you for a soft drink, a shot of whiskey, or a juicy steak. So, what do most Americans do when they're thirsty? They put the absolutely wrong things into their bodies.

Second, look in the mirror. As the popular television psychologist would ask, "How's that standard American diet working for you?" We've got to logically conclude that what we as a society are dumping into our bodies is wrong. Something is just not working despite all the media hype. It's not helping us live a healthy life. As a matter of fact, the foods we ingest are hurting us in more ways than I can count.

Third, truth does exist. But, it is not necessarily where you would expect to find it. While I agree with many of the professionals out there, I want to go one step further. Yes, I'll talk about high fructose corn syrup, preservatives, and the toxins in the world. But where did the ideas about healthy living originate in the first place? Who set the standard? Who created what I call the heart of health?

You see, I want to help you understand the reason you have a health problem and then help you find the ultimate solution and not merely how to treat a symptom. The answers include much more than the foods you eat or the time you spend immobile in front of TV screens or computer monitors.

It also includes the thoughts you think, who or what you worship, and how willing you are to love and be loved.

The answers, my friend, exist. This is the journey I traveled with David. However, I needed to move slowly, one step at a time.

The Journey

Once David was out of immediate danger, I had a chance to sit down with him and try to explain exactly what he'd been through.

Blockage of the arteries supplying the heart with blood is termed "coronary artery disease," or simply CAD. The problem develops because the coronary arteries become narrowed or completely blocked by plaque. When this occurs, blood, with its life-sustaining supply of oxygen, can't reach the heart muscle. Without oxygen, the heart begins to "suffocate" and will eventually stop pumping.

What causes the arteries to be clogged? Your body carries fats called lipids in the blood. Lipids can gradually build up inside the blood vessels. These buildups can become hardened or calcified. Then other elements become involved, making the blockages bigger and unstable. Blood has an increasingly difficult time passing through the arteries. This was the situation David was in when he was rushed to the hospital. He was experiencing an acute problem needing immediate acute care.

One thing to keep in mind is plaque buildup can be occurring in any artery anywhere in the body, including the brain, aorta, or legs. Developing hand in hand with this buildup is inflammation within the arteries.

Sometimes a blockage, which is also called a "plaque mat," can become unstable. If this mat, which I sometimes think of as a "pimple," pops, there could be big problems even if there's only a 30-40 percent narrowing in the artery. The body sees this rupture as an injury and sends what it believes to be healing cells to the site.

If you cut your arm, many different types of cells are recruited to fight the damage. The same thing happens inside the artery when a plaque mat ruptures. These cells, rushing to the rescue, mean to do us good, and that's usually what they do. But at the mat rupture site, they may do something less than helpful. They finish plugging up what little open space remains in the artery. The result? Blood flow is stopped and the owner of the artery experiences a debilitating heart attack.

How many of us are going through life thinking everything is just fine when, unseen and unfelt, something is building inside of us—something dangerous and life threatening?

I went on to explain to David that, unfortunately, at this time in history, there are no diagnostic tests to predict which plaques will rupture. If we had this test, we could predict heart attacks. We can, however, predict which people are at a greater risk. When David's plaque "popped," the recruited damage-fighting cells formed a clot, resulting in a great restriction of blood flow in the artery. Severe pain caused by a heart muscle not receiving enough blood immediately followed.

The cornerstone in the acute treatment of CAD is first to restore blood flow to the heart as quickly as possible. Time lost is muscle lost. If blood flow is not restored quickly by opening the blocked artery, permanent damage to the heart will occur. Because of the lack of blood flow to the heart, the body's electrical system could be damaged and malfunction, resulting in a dangerously slow, fast, or uneven heart rhythm. When these rhythms occur, the heart may not be able to pump sufficient blood to the other organs of the body, and these organs also can begin to malfunction. This is exactly what happened to David.

In addition, the heart valves controlling the direction of blood flow depend on muscles that may be damaged during a heart attack. So, now you've got blood flowing, but in the wrong direction!

Most severe of all, during a heart attack, it's even possible that a dead heart muscle may break open or rupture. This situation is usually fatal.

David shook his head in utter amazement. He'd felt nothing until that attack. He didn't know it was coming. "So, Doctor Marcum," he said. "This plaque, where did it come from?"

There are times in life when the truth bites like a lion. This was one of those times. "David," I said, "the stressors in your life, including the cigarettes you smoked, the foods you ate, and the genetics bombs you triggered with your lifestyle, caused this to happen."

Sources
Remember when I mentioned lipids a few paragraphs back? Lipids are the fats that create plaque. What I didn't mention was where they came from.

A lipid is an oily, organic compound insoluble in water that, along with proteins and carbohydrates, is an essential structural component of every living cell. In other words, lipids are good. Your cells need them to be a cell.

These fats need to be ingested. In our diet, there are two sources of lipids— animal products and plant products. Both deliver fat to the body. So, we supply our bodies with lipids each time we eat.

But, here's the problem. Animal products contain high levels of fat. As a matter of fact, some products such as cheese are almost entirely fat.

Plant foods, on the other hand, are very low in fat, providing just enough for cell development and maintenance. So, when I toss out a statistic such as "It has been estimated up to 80 percent of heart attacks before the age of 65 could be prevented," one of the main elements driving that statistic is diet.

Think of all the lives that could be saved if people understood what I just said. But they don't know. Why? Because the meat industry is a multibillion-dollar conglomeration able to mount incredibly expensive advertising campaigns that convince us meat is good for us, that milk is good for us, that pork is good for us.

When was the last time you watched a "Carrots are good for you" commercial on television? When was the last time you heard the words "Where's the spinach?" so often that it became a cultural catchphrase? When was the last time you read in a popular magazine an ad headlining the words "Got soy?"

Excess fat in the body, just like excess tension, excess guilt, excess stimulation of any kind, stresses the organs, including the heart. These stresses can be totally hidden, working unseen and unfelt deep inside us, causing our systems to malfunction and, as in David's case, almost shut down entirely.

The concept of food as a stressor may be a new thought for many. It was to David. All those hamburgers; all those deep-fried fries; all those juicy steaks and barbecued ribs; all those creamy bowls of ice cream and frosty glasses of milk placed unseen and unfelt stresses on his body as they provided the building blocks for a steady buildup of plaque. Then came the tipping point with unbearable pain and a race to the hospital. Now he had his stent. The blood was flowing again. But the problem wasn't fixed.

Let's be practical for a moment. If you begin to feel symptoms you cannot explain; if you think you are having a heart attack, here's what you need to do. Don't ignore the feeling. Sit down, call 911, and leave the phone off the hook so your call can be traced just in case you get too weak to talk or pass out. If possible, take an aspirin and try your best to relax. DO NOT drive yourself to the emergency room.

If a friend or neighbor, instead of an ambulance, takes you to the hospital, let everyone know when you arrive that you think you're having a heart attack. This is no time to sit down in the waiting room and wait your turn. If you are having feelings you cannot explain, the sooner you seek help the better.

David was very, very fortunate. But his journey was far from over.

Chapter 3

Asking Why

The numbers are staggering. Researchers at the National Coalition on Health Care believe that by 2017, health care may account for $4.3 trillion in annual spending—a fifth of every dollar needed to keep our economy running.

Right now the direct and indirect cost for smoking rings in at $193 billion per year according to the Centers for Disease Control and Prevention. Diabetes cost this country $116 billion in 2007 and heart disease lifted $305 billion from the nation's coffers in 2009 for acute services, medications, and lost productivity. Obesity? Our girth isn't the only thing that's being supersized. Treating this condition and the cascade of diseases for which it opens doors is draining $147 billion annually from our collective savings accounts. These are just estimates of the rising expense of health care.

But money really is not the issue for me. It's the tears I see in so many eyes, the distorted sounds that echo in my stethoscope, the troubling images emerging from MRIs, CAT scans, and X-ray machines that create the greatest concern in my mind. People are suffering, and in so many cases, the suffering is self-imposed; not from lives lived in defiance of sound health laws, but from ignorance of them. David was just such a case.

During my follow-up visits with him, I began to realize something interesting. When it comes to knowing how to properly care for the human body, my own search for truth was, in many ways, paralleling his search.

Medical school had done a terrific job of preparing me for the most effective ways to treat acute illnesses. I'd become very adept at keeping people alive using the amazing tools of the cardiology trade. I could diagnose a heart problem very rapidly and apply the needed technology to keep my patient's family from cashing in on his or her life insurance policy. But as I began to see my patients returning to me with the very same conditions time and time again, I realized my training had not gone far enough. I'd become a doctor to make people well, not just keep them from dying.

Many years ago when I was a medical resident, I helped take care of a man with a malignancy. The medical team in charge of his care thought a bone marrow transplant was the way to go. So we began blasting him with powerful chemotherapy to kill the malignant cells. As is usually the case with chemotherapy, this also killed off many of his good cells. I remember watching his white and red blood cell count drop as his bone marrow succumbed to the powerful chemotherapy. We had to give him blood transfusions to keep the red blood cells up and then load him up with various antibiotics at the faintest sign of infection because he had too few white blood cells, which thwart infections.

The man suffered greatly under the treatment. The medications made him sick. He was nauseated most of the time. But our patient was courageous, even though he was isolated in a sterile room, could see his family only for limited periods, and was constantly bombarded with the best modern medicine had to offer.

Soon it was time for the marrow transplant. Hopes ran high that the malignancy was gone. Yes, he was gaining strength, but the strain on his system had left him looking much older than his age. While I was amazed at the science and technology that surrounded the case, deep down I felt something was missing. Our hopes, the family's hopes, our patient's hopes were all tied into what modern medicine could do—and I was part of that. What if modern medicine failed to work?

Not long after the marrow transplant, my patient became desperately ill. A sudden infection gripped his body in a terrible embrace and, despite the application of a ventilator, dialysis, and intravenous medications and nutrition, he died.

As he was nearing the end, I was in his room caring for him. I remember him looking at me with unspoken questions in his eyes, but he passed away before I could provide any answers. I wanted to reach out to him with hope, but did not have the words to say. This bothered me a great deal. Everything I knew—everything modern medicine had to offer—was not enough to save him. That's when I turned to God with that same look in my eyes. There had to be more—more information, more insights, more truth than what I had been taught in medical school. Right then and there I prayed for God to open my eyes to truth and give me the courage to speak out even if others were silent.

A slow journey began that continues to this day. I started looking beyond my medical textbooks for answers. I ultimately began searching for healing truth where most people search for spiritual truth—in the pages of God's Holy Word. And what I found was astonishing.

The Question Why

The first thing I did in my search for understanding of disease was to begin asking the all-important and often overlooked question "Why?" Why is this heart sick? Why is this person short of breath? Why is my patient suffering such debilitating pain? Why does a disease that just a few years ago attacked only the elderly challenge this young person? Why does the human body react this way or that way? Why are cardiovascular diseases, diabetes, obesity, and cancer rates soaring to such incredible heights? We were not created to be sick. Experiencing a heart attack was not part of the original plan God had in mind for His created beings.

I wanted something concrete—something unchanging upon which to attach my mode of operation as a physician.

It became painfully obvious to me that I was being deceived into thinking that understanding why is not important. I soon realized others are being deceived as well. Voices keep telling us truth does not matter; we should simply let someone else tell us how or what to think. We're being told to let the television, radio, or the Internet think for us. If a doctor or preacher says it, it *must* be true. You don't need to understand why things happen. Just accept them as inevitable facts of life and go on as best you can.

But those same voices keep tripping over themselves. "This medicine is great," I hear them proclaim. Then just as my patients are almost adjusted to that particular brand's side effects, I read about it being pulled off the market—something about people dying.

"Low fat is good," I hear. Then the next month, "High carb is the way to go!"

"Caffeine is good."

"Caffeine is bad."

In our heavily marketed world, how does one know who or what to believe? Allow me to be brutally honest. Too many people are making money at the expense of others. Our good health is not the driving force behind many products today. Our ignorance is. Unscrupulous companies are depending on our being too uninformed or simply too busy to discover the truth. In essence, we are being held captive by our own lack of interest in the question "Why?"

One of the first Bible texts that caught my attention as I began studying into that very question was this gem: "You will know the truth, and the truth will set you free" (John 8:32). That is exactly what I wanted. I wanted to be free from hype and tradition. I wanted my interaction with patients to be based on healing advice, not profitable prescriptions. While I was certainly ready to deal with any acute condition that came my way, I wanted to make sure when my patient left my office, he or she would have real information that could be used to deal effectively with their condition over the long haul. I did not want my patient back to see me in a few months suffering from a new malady brought on by the same old condition on which I'd placed a bandage. I wanted him or her cured. Yes, I wanted their problem *fixed*.

Stress as Cause

Emily is 64 years old. Her children are grown and married, living in different states. But her life is far from peaceful. Her 86-year-old mother is suffering from Alzheimer's disease, and Emily has been the woman's sole caregiver for the past five years. Daily, she feeds her mother, bathes her, gives her medications, points out the date, and even explains to her time and time again that, yes, she is her daughter.

For the past three years, Emily has given up most of her social life and her marriage has suffered because she spends the bulk of her time in the caregiver mold. Unfortunately, the family does not possess the resources to utilize a special-care facility.

What Emily—and the thousands like her facing this type of situation—doesn't realize is her stressful life could very well be changing the chemical environment within her own body. This chronic stress could cause any number of illnesses. That's right. The life Emily is living could make her very, very sick.

The dictionary defines stress as the physical, chemical, or emotional factor that causes bodily or mental tension and may be a factor in disease causation. Originally, we were designed by God to live totally stress free—no selfishness, no disease, no clueless bosses or unrepentant enemies, no wayward children or disenfranchised spouses, no having to explain to your own mother who you are. We were created to live in a perfect, love-filled world.

As time advanced, we had greater and greater stressors placed on our bodies. Now we even have to carry the heavy genetic load of stress passed down to us from previous generations. Add to that polluted environments, toxic foods, and information overload and you can see how far we have drifted from the original stress-free plan.

The body's response to stress can involve more than 1,400 chemical reactions utilizing up to 30 different hormones and neurotransmitters. These are just the reactions we know about!

We've all heard of the stress hormone epinephrine, also called adrenaline. When we are under stress, the body releases this chemical, which places us in the so-called fight-or-flight mode. This is not necessarily a bad thing. If you saw a rattlesnake in the road, ready to strike, adrenaline would kick in and you'd jump back. We've all heard the stories of supernatural strength occurring in stressful situations when the body is pumping out adrenaline at high levels.

Epinephrine is released by the adrenal glands. A sister hormone is norepinephrine. When these chemicals are released, nerves throughout the body—using something called the "sympathetic nervous system"—are activated. What occurs next is a miracle. Your heart rate increases as needed. Your heart pumps more blood, rushing increased levels of oxygen to the body. Your blood vessels constrict, diverting needed blood to your muscles and brain and away from your skin and digestive tract. Under these extreme and temporary conditions, your muscles can do more, lift more, and react faster. Your brain is quicker, too, reaching conclusions rapidly on how to address the problem. Your pupils dilate so you can see better—even in low-light situations. Sugars and fats are moved into your blood to supply added energy. Your blood clots faster in case there is bleeding. Your brain becomes very focused.

But there is more. Cortisol is released, which stimulates the delivery of fuel for energy. Cortisol is usually secreted in a 24-hour pattern, highest in the morning and lowest around midnight. But in times of stress, it's made available in high amounts *right now*.

As I said, this is all fine and good if there's a rattlesnake in your path. But, we as a society seem to have a lot more than poisonous snakes getting in our way. We've got bumper-to-bumper traffic, psychotic coworkers, rude neighbors, demanding bosses, and disrespectful children. Our fight-or-flight mode is switched on almost constantly. That means all of the special functions I listed above can be engaged constantly. That's just not good for a body. More to the point, that's just not healthy.

When the body is under chronic stress from whatever the cause, cortisol levels, for instance, remain elevated. If these levels are high at night, sleep is disturbed, the body cannot rest, and more stress is added to the system. High levels of cortisol cause extra insulin production and the body responds to this by *storing* fat instead of burning fat. Extra fat, sometimes called the endocannabinoid system, generates its own hormones and chemical environment, which puts more stress on the body. Inflammation can be stimulated. Chronic inflammation, in turn, is a stressor leading to many dangerous conditions, including heart disease.

The point I'm trying to make is acute stress and its chemical reactions are a needed response from time to time. But chronic stress damages the system via a host of chemical reactions involving the entire body—the mind, the cardiovascular system, even metabolism. In short, our entire being is impacted by the chronic stress under which we all seem to be living with these days. So there's little wonder that we're facing skyrocketing rates of obesity, diabetes, high blood pressure, heart attacks, irregular heart rhythms, insomnia, infections (stress chemistry weakens the immune system), depression, inflammation, and the list goes on and on and on. All can be traced to the chemistry of chronic stress.

The Sad Truth

The sad truth is the world—including the health-care industry—does not relieve a state of chronic stress. No one goes around saying this out loud, but think about it. There is a lot more money to be made from sick people than from well people. Remove stress, and you remove the cause of most diseases. No chronic stress means no need for all those pills, potions, doctor visits, surgeries, therapy sessions, and endless research that addresses the results of being stressed out.

This thought formed a turning point in my career. Instead of chasing after symptoms, I decided discovering what was stressing the system was the best way to really make people whole again. If I knew why they were sick, I could do much more good than simply trying to make them comfortable in their sickness.

Did it ever cross my mind that if I taught my patients how not to get sick, they would not need me anymore? Certainly. But I also knew it is human nature to resist change—even if the change is ultimately good for you. There would always be people who refused to change, and I wanted to be there for them, too. But for those willing to follow my lead, they could begin making real changes in their lives—changes that would reduce or eliminate their need for modern medicine.

So, when David stepped into my office for our next follow-up visit, I was ready for him. Like it or not, I was going to find out what was stressing his system, and then teach him how to eliminate all possible stressors. My goal was to, eventually, not ever have to see him again—as his doctor.

Chapter 4

Hidden Stresses

D avid, do you take a shower every day?"
My patient stared pensively at me for a moment. "Yes, Doctor Marcum," he said, squirming uneasily in his chair. "Is there a reason you asked that particular question?"

I laughed. "No. You're very clean."

"Are you suggesting taking a daily shower is a good treatment for heart disease?"

"Well, not exactly," I said, "although it would probably improve many people's social lives. I just wanted to observe your response so I could ask yet another question. How do you feel if you miss a shower for a day or two?"

David grinned shyly. "Smelly. Grungy."

I folded my patient's chart and placed it carefully on my desk. "The point I'm trying to make is there are certain things we need to do daily in order to accomplish something important. For instance, you shower every day to stay clean and not offend anyone with body odor, right?"

"Right."

"And it's probably safe for me to say you use water for your shower instead of, oh, maybe, soda pop or honey."

David nodded. "I try to stay away from cranberry juice and gasoline, too."

"Right," I chuckled. "You use water because water is the only substance that really cleans the human body. Add a touch of soap, perhaps a rubber ducky, and you're good to go. Squeaky-clean. No odor. All because of water."

My patient eyed me suspiciously. "Something tells me there's a broader direction in this conversation."

I picked up his chart again and started slowly and deliberately leafing through it. "Can I be honest with you?" I asked.

"I would not expect anything else from the man who helped save my life.

Fire away!"

I paused and studied my patient for a long drawn-out moment. "David, you have been taking better care of your outside than your inside. You always come into my office dressed in clean clothes; hair combed, teeth brushed, shoes shined. Yet through the years, you have been ignoring what's inside. Outside, you look great. Inside, there are unseen problems."

David frowned. "What do you mean?"

"Well, let's stay with water. When was the last time you enjoyed a great big glass of pure, unadulterated water just because you wanted to? Is there a big water jug in your refrigerator at home waiting to quench your thirst? Do you carry a water bottle around with you just in case you get a little parched on the job?"

David shook his head. "Water is boring," he said. "Who drinks that?"

"Not very many people," I responded. "As a matter of fact, it's been estimated up to 70 percent of us Americans are dehydrated. And in that condition, an amazing amount of stress is brought to your body. Your heart works harder. Your blood is thicker. Your brain doesn't think as clearly. Because of the lack of water your kidneys are working overtime trying to filter out impurities from your blood. Your intestines and colon are bogged down, filled with byproducts of digestion without a proper solution of water and fiber to move the waste material along. The stress chemistry is turned on when it is not needed. I could go on and on, but my point is all of these problems are associated directly with the fact that you are not drinking enough water."

"So, if I drink more water, my heart problem will go away?"

"It's certainly a step in the right direction, but there's more. A lot more."

As a doctor, I am always challenged to find ways of getting my patients to see the bigger picture when it comes to their health. It all comes down to stress—stress on the organs, stress on the brain, stress on the blood supply, stress on the heart. Many times, my patients do not even realize they are bringing almost unbearable stress upon their bodies. Stress is often the hidden cause of disease leading to symptoms and the need for my services. Stress is indeed a hidden danger. Let me explain.

It is common knowledge today that smoking—and secondhand smoke— is a huge source of chronic stress on the human physiology. But many still smoke. Inadequate rest produces enormous amounts of stress as well, yet we're sleeping about two hours less per night than our great-grandfathers did.

Most do not take a day off. It's a 24/7 world we live in.

Then there's our environment. We're filling our homes with smells we were never designed to sample. Synthetic perfumes and "lightly scented" toiletries and laundry soaps are introducing into our bodies elements that are—to be blunt—poison.

We take perfectly good foods and process the nutrients right out of them, leaving a bland and colorless product requiring copious amounts of additives such as salt and sugar to make them even palatable. We put trans fats and high fructose corn syrup sprinkled with chemicals our body does not know how to handle into all the most convenient foods. What we can't process, we ignore. Then we wonder why we do not have energy, so we slosh down another cup of coffee.

Being overweight also brings an incredible amount of stress to the human body. Again the stress chemistry is activated. Here's an interesting point to ponder. As we gain weight, we do not gain structure. The very same bones supporting a 160-pound man are called on to support him when he weighs 360 pounds. No, we weren't designed to be fat. If we are overweight, we are placing added and unneeded stress on a system that might already be overwhelmed. Yet obesity rates are hovering at dangerous levels. The numbers continue to rise.

Consider our delicate digestive system. It accepts food, extracts the needed nutrients, makes energy available to the muscles, and basically fuels our lives. But we often keep dumping fuel into our system exactly when we do not need it—in the evening before we go to bed. Then we don't fuel ourselves exactly when we need it most—in the morning before we head off to work.

Even water, the all-important ingredient keeping us healthy, has become the beverage no one orders at a restaurant. If a waiter happens to place a glass in front of us, we might allow our dehydrated bodies a few sips before turning our attention to our favorite soda pop or alcoholic drink—both of which actually can serve as a diuretic and remove water from our system. The same water, the universal solvent, that cleans us so well on the outside is the perfect beverage to clean us on the inside, yet we ignore it and call it boring. Remember, up to 70 percent of the body is made of water. It is the most important ingredient.

When it comes to our minds, we are not being all too diligent there either. A bad work environment, memories we cannot seem to escape, unrelenting anger, soul-scarring grief, unresolved guilt, and endless loneliness all work in concert to add extreme stress to our whole being. Toss in a couple divorces, sour relationships, and a life dependent on a bank's credit line and, well, look around at the crowded doctors' offices and pharmacies and you get the picture. These hidden stresses are sucking the health right out of our minds and bodies, filling them instead with the valueless junk of fast food, fast times, and fast-working diseases. Our illnesses aren't killing us. *We're* killing us. Disease is often just a symptom of a life being lived out of step with the reality of how we were designed to live.

"There you go again," David said as I returned to my seat behind my desk. "Designed to live. *Designed to live.* How can we know how we were designed to live? We weren't made in a factory somewhere. We didn't come with an owner's manual."

"That's where you're wrong, David," I said as gently as I could. "I know exactly where we came from and, yes, we do have an owner's manual. But few talk, preach, or sing about it. It is not considered high tech or on the cutting edge to make this part of a treatment plan. It has to be one of the best-kept secrets in the world."

David looked at me skeptically. "OK, Doc," he said. "Write me a prescription for it and I'll pick it up on my way home. It is covered by my medical plan, right?"

I smiled. "Tell you what," I said as I walked my patient to the door. "During our next visit, I'll give you a manual free. No charge."

My patient blinked. "A doctor giving out free meds? This I gotta see."

As I watched David walk down the hall, I thought pensively about our conversation. Throughout time, physicians have wanted to blame one agent or the other as the possible cause of illness and cardiovascular disease. Eating the wrong foods, cigarettes, and more recently high cholesterol levels have been implicated. Physicians are now looking at inflammation as a possible smoking gun. I wish it were that simple. I wish I could say to someone, "Your genetics say you will get heart disease, so you may as well start taking medications such as the statins to lower your cholesterol. As a matter of fact, let's just put statins in our water supply so everyone is safe." Don't laugh. It's been discussed.

Besides making a few pharmaceutical companies very, very happy—and even richer than they are now—such a radical approach to heart disease would do little to stem the tide. Heart disease is still the number one killer in the country in spite of the fact we have been doling out powerful medicines and have developed complex procedures and devices designed to combat it for years. The bottom line is *stress* on the system causes heart disease—the chronic stressors we allow into our lives that build up until our bodies are overwhelmed with adverse chemistry. This stress can come from many different sources and is on the rise in the world we live in. This stress can be cumulative. Then a symptom develops. Sometimes, tragically, the first symptom is a full-blown heart attack. This was the case with David.

While some of my patients suffer from purely genetic stress problems such as congenital abnormalities, including bad heart valves, certain abnormal heart rhythms, and even weak hearts, most cardiovascular disease is acquired. When we put chronic stress on the system, damage occurs, and then we look to modern medicine to bring us back from the brink. Sometimes it can, often it can't.

In today's world, it's not only the patient's heart that's broken. It's our health system as well.

Perpetuating Illness

If I were trying to perpetuate illness in the world, I would sneak in just enough truth in the popular media and modern medical practices to make it believable, add some good marketing techniques to convince people modern medicine can cure their ills, and then make my fortune treating symptoms with expensive pills and procedures. Next I would throw in some special medicines that numb the senses just enough to make people think their problem is solved. I would try to figure out techniques to get people to turn to other people—or even the government—for truth. I would use the media to control minds and discourage patients from thinking or asking questions. I'd encourage society to be too busy—even doing good things—to think at all.

Then I would convince religious denominations to become politically active machines, bent on preserving certain belief systems by urging members to become judgmental, legalistic, and overly indoctrinated. When it comes to health care, I would have impressive and sophisticated high-tech devices and treatments delivered by intelligent people.

In the natural world, I would encourage folk to look to certain foods, nutraceuticals, specific herbs, or some New Age theory as a cure for *all* problems, using the power of the Internet to present and support my claims.

Finally, I would slowly poison the people with taste-pleasing foods— foods that destroy the environment during their production. I'd encourage everyone to exhaust themselves, making the fast-paced, grab-it-while-you-can, everything-all-the-time lifestyle the ultimate goal. Then, I would sprinkle in a few wars, natural disasters, new taxes, and be on my way. Lastly, I would never want people to ask "Why?"

The horror of it all is, what I just described is exactly what is happening in this world today. Illness is being perpetuated. It's precisely the mode of operation of some unseen, unrecognized power moving among us like a dark shadow. I promised David a free prescription for his heart disease. I had to deliver on my promise. After months of searching for answers, I felt I had something to offer. He'd asked for an owner's manual for his body. I was bound and determined to give him one.

Chapter 5

Deadly Deceptions

We have a big problem in this country—a serious, life-threatening problem. And part of the problem is coming from the very industry on which we depend during our times of illness.

I am a medical doctor—a board-certified cardiologist to be exact. I use very powerful medications and procedures to treat acute cases every day. Without the proper administration of these pharmaceuticals and procedures, many of my patients could die.

The problem originates from the strong belief that these medications contain healing powers. At best, they have the ability to sidetrack a problem; to work around it in order to keep a person alive long enough to enable actual healing to occur. When administered properly, medications and procedures can do some pretty amazing things. They definitely have the ability to improve symptoms.

It is when you move out of the emergency room, out of the acute care setting, that drugs can become anything but your best friend. Here you uncover a deception that, if fully identified, would put some people in jail.

Let me ask you a few pointed questions. How often do you leave a doctor's office with a new prescription tucked neatly in your purse or wallet? How often do you stand in line at the drugstore, waiting for a magic paper sack containing what your physician says will deal effectively with your latest ailment? How much did you—and your health insurance plan—pay for that paper sack?

For all the money you just spent; for all the training your doctor underwent; for all the safeguards built into the pharmaceutical system imposed by our very own Food and Drug Administration (FDA), you would think what you were about to drop down your throat or inject into your skin would be entirely safe. Think again.

According to Mike Adams, a consumer health advocate, "The entire drug industry, including the monopolistic drug giants and their FDA coconspirator, has clearly become the single greatest threat to the health and safety of the American people. And yet the FDA continues to push more drugs onto more Americans than ever before, all the while pretending these drugs are safe and effective when, in reality, they are neither." Look at the ads on the television or in the print media and you will see what I mean.

The Centers for Disease Control and Prevention (CDC) provides numbers that seem to back up Mr. Adams' rather startling claims. In its Morbidity and Mortality Weekly Report released in 2007, researchers reported "deaths from prescription drugs rose from 4.4 per 100,000 people in 1999 to 7.1 per 100,000 in 2004. This increase represents a jump from 11,000 people to almost 20,000 in the span of five years. Among the 20,000 who died, more than 8,500— double the number from 1999—were from 'other and unspecified drugs.' Psychotherapeutic drugs, like antidepressants and sedatives, nearly doubled from 671 deaths to 1,300."

In a landmark study released in 2003 entitled "Death by Medicine," authors Gary Null, Ph.D., Carolyn Dean, M.D., Martin Feldman, M.D., Debora Rasio, M.D., and Dorothy Smith, Ph.D., added fuel to the fire. "A definitive review and close reading of medical peer-review journals, and government health statistics shows that American medications frequently cause more harm than good. . . . The number of people having in-hospital, adverse drug reactions (ADR) to prescribed medicine is 2.2 million. Dr. Richard Besser, of the CDC, in 1995, said the number of unnecessary antibiotics prescribed annually for viral infections was 20 million. Dr. Besser, in 2003, now refers to tens of millions of unnecessary antibiotics. The number of unnecessary medical and surgical procedures performed annually is 7.5 million. The number of people exposed to unnecessary hospitalization annually is 8.9 million. The total number of iatrogenic [inadvertent physician-induced] deaths . . . is 783,936. It is evident that it is entirely possible the American medical system could be the leading cause of death and injury in the United States. The 2001 heart disease annual death rate is 699,697; the annual cancer death rate, 553,251." Since this study was released, the situation has only gotten worse.

According to these numbers, you could be more likely to die from the treatment than from the disease. Yet we continue to spend billions of dollars each year seeking cures by prescription. Something is terribly wrong. It is not completely the fault of the doctors, hospitals, drug companies, and other health-care providers. The users or consumers, that's you and me, want a quick fix, and often do not want to find and treat the cause, which is ultimately the best solution.

So, who is going to fix the problem, or is the problem even fixable? I doubt it will be our governmental agencies. There are far too many lobbyists, too much red tape, too much politicking, and big companies willing to donate enormous amounts of money to those in power. How about the media? Not likely, too many advertising dollars to be collected. Physicians? Who wants the hassle—and the criticism? Maybe our attorneys? Nope. Medical lawsuits earn them millions each year.

That leaves you and me—the ordinary citizen. But first, we have to recognize the deception, know where it came from, and how best to overturn its influence in our lives. Until we do this, we remain victims of our own ignorance.

Again, let me say some medications and treatments are always needed, especially for acute life-threatening situations. But all produce stress on the human body. We were just not designed for them, and I have not yet used a medication that did not have a side effect. Risks versus benefits must constantly be weighed. For instance, knowing fully that antibiotics have no effect on viruses, doctors are writing endless prescriptions for antibiotics because patients are demanding them for viral infections. The microorganisms are becoming more drug resistant. Why are they becoming drug resistant? Because of all the antibiotics we're taking.

We are overprescribing acid-blocking medications. Stomach acid is a great defense against unwanted bacterial "bugs." And patients on these acid-blocking medications can double their chance of developing pneumonia and diarrhea. These commonly prescribed medications—as well as their over-the-counter cousins—also decrease calcium absorption, thus tripling the risk of hip fractures. Yet many of these same medications boast "calcium added" in their promotions. They have included the very thing their presence interrupts.

What about sleeping pills? Those who take them regularly can experience a fivefold increase in cognitive defects along with more daytime fatigue. Those pills knock you out but do not provide the needed rest.

This list could go on to include memory pills, pain pills, and some diabetes prescriptions. I think you get the picture. Drugs are not always what they seem to be. Then there are those who take them for "recreational or escape" purposes.

So what do we do? What do I as a physician do? That is the very question I asked myself years ago as I began to realize what I was doing for people was not helping them in the long run. I was keeping them alive long enough for their disease or condition to regroup and attack again. This was a great *business* plan, but I knew something "big" was missing.

An Answer

I was born and raised a Christian. I attended church, sang hymns, read my Bible, and prayed. I tried to connect with God. But, for some reason, I never connected worship to health. More to the point, I never connected worship to the *building and maintaining* of health. Christianity was something I did, something I believed, not something I utilized to stay healthy.

All this changed dramatically when I began to see a convergence taking place; a coming together of two elements—biblical truths and science. As scientists gained the tools necessary to peer further and further into what makes life possible, I found that my faithful Bible began to make more sense. It was as if modern researchers were seeking and discovering the proofs to verify what my Bible teaches. Study after study seemed to emphasize certain biblical passages, bringing to light their ancient truths. This merging of science and the Bible changed the way I regarded Scripture and launched me on a search for healing and the practice of medicine that continues to this day. I realized, at this point in history, science was not refuting biblical truth; it was actually proving it!

Health and good chemistry were not just about eating the right foods and getting sufficient exercise. They were not just about pills versus plants or organic versus conventional. Many treatments are out there for every condition known to humans, but there was something much more important needing to be emphasized.

In my own search for truth, I came to realize true health is actually a by-product, an end result, of a love relationship with God. It begins with Him loving us, and ends with us loving Him. Everything else—every choice we make, every habit we overcome, every thought we think—must be a direct result of that growing connection we enjoy with the One who created us.

Follow me closely for a moment. The further we move away from that connection, the sicker we become, and the more stress is put on the system. Originally we were designed to worship God and become like what we worship. For optimal health and well-being, it's essential to know the Great Physician. This is the way we were made to operate. When we worship anything else— money, power, technology, modern medicine, food, sports, movie stars, religious institutions, television, the Internet (the list goes on and on)—we move away from the original plan and stress chemistry appears. This type of worship was not in the original design. I knew that in order to help David find real, lasting healing, I would have to connect him with worship of the God he was designed to know, along with the lifestyle he was created to follow.

Our next meeting would be critical to his long-term healing process.

Second Chances

It was obvious to me David was improving. By following simple suggestions concerning diet and exercise, his chemistry was changing right before my eyes. He had lost a little weight, his cholesterol was edging downward, his energy was improving, he slept better at night, and his heartbeat sounded stronger and more regular in my stethoscope. His blood pressure was heading back into the normal range and the pungent smell of cigarette smoke was barely noticeable now. I made a few notations on his chart and then studied him thoughtfully.

"So," he said with a smile, "how'm I doin'?"

"You're doing well," I said. "But I want to remind you that—"

"I know. I'm not fixed. I'm just patched. I've got more work to do."

I smiled. "You've been listening to me. I'm flattered!"

David grinned. "Hey, our conversation here a month ago was kind of a wake-up call. I figure I've been given a second chance."

"I agree," I said, sitting down beside my patient. "And that's why I've got something for you. You can call it your "second chance kit.""

"Oh, yeah," David beamed. "My free meds! I was hoping you hadn't forgotten."

I reached into a drawer in a nearby cabinet and withdrew a small, rectangular package. "Here you go. Take two of these and call me in the morning."

Like a child at Christmas, David quickly ripped open the packaging, then paused. "A Bible?" he exclaimed. "You're giving me a Bible?" He seemed

THE HEART OF HEALTH: AVOIDING DECEPTION

disappointed.

"Good medicine," I said.

"Doc, I don't mean to sound ungrateful, but I'm not what you'd call a Christian. Bibles are for Christians, right?"

"Really?" I said. "The Bible is good for everybody. Christians have simply figured that out already."

My patient thought for a moment. "I . . . ah . . ."

"Listen, David," I said, learning forward in my chair. "God did not say what He said in this Book because we love Him. He said what He said because He loves us. And because He loves us, He created laws that make life possible— and that includes, for example, the various laws of physics. You jump off a building; you're going to fall. That's the law of gravity in full operation whether or not you believe in it, or the God who created it.

"Well, that same God who created the law of gravity created a rather precise collection of laws pertaining directly to our health. Break a science law and something bad usually happens. Break a health law and you get sick. Your chemistry gets messed up. You stress the body. It's as simple as that."

"How do I know the words in that black Book are really true? How do I know those writings are not just an elaborate way the world has developed to cope with the inevitable, death?" David questioned. "That is a great and relevant question," I responded. I explained to him that God spoke His message to us through mere humans, about 40 writers, from about 1100 B.C. to around 100 years after the birth of Christ. These were His spokespersons.

Again, David asked, "How do I know without doubt the words they spoke were from the God of the universe?"

"Well," I explained, "you could look at all the fulfilled prophecies; events predicted hundreds of years ahead of time. History shows all these events came to pass—from the rise of kingdoms like the Greek and Roman empires predicted in the book of Daniel to the birth of Christ foretold in great detail in the book of Isaiah. History has proven the Bible to be true—from the Dead Sea scrolls, which contain fragments of many Bible books, to archaeological finds still being unearthed today. Science, as illustrated by the concepts in this Book, validates the Bible.

"David," I continued, "read the book *More Than a Carpenter,* by Josh McDowell. This helped me when I needed proof that the Bible was true. I had similar questions."

I then added that what helped me most was something a wise person said to me during my searching moments. "'Don't let other people think for you. You can read all the material out there. You can talk to the most educated people from both camps. But, what I suggest is this: Give God a chance to prove that the Bible is true. Get a Bible and begin to read. Ask God to show you if this Book is truly His words or fiction. If you have an open mind and are sincere in your search, you will receive an answer.'

"This is the path I took, David. As I began to communicate with God, He began to talk to me and show me truth. The first truth was that I could depend on Him. When I did this, I could see Him leading in the events of my life. He was showing me not only that the Bible was true, but that He loved me and wanted to be a part of my life."

In a world where it's tough to know who or what to believe, I found the answer. I soon discovered the Bible also gives guidelines on the prevention and treatment of disease. When applied, these principles change the chemistry much like a pill or procedure without the side effects and address the cause of the problem. In today's world this type of thinking is missing. Conversely, when these biblical principles are violated, we damage the body's fabric. I want my children, Kelli and Jake, to be healthy and make good decisions because I love them and want them to be happy. God gives us suggestions in the Bible for the same reason. He loves us and wants us to be happy. The Creator is the real Master Physician, the one I want to listen to first.

David stiffened. "So, you're saying I had a heart attack because I was breaking some of God's laws? Well, excuse me. I thought you told me I had my heart attack because I was smoking, eating too much fatty food, and not getting enough exercise. Where is it written: 'Thou shalt not smoke, eat junk food, or sit on your butt all day'?"

"I'm glad you asked that question, David," I said as I lifted the Bible from my patient's hand and turned to the very first pages. "If it's OK with you, I'd like to read you a story. And when we're finished, you tell me why you had a heart attack."

David looked at me skeptically, then glanced down at the Bible as I began to read.

Chapter 6

In the Beginning

When I began to write this book, the Holy Spirit impressed me to write in a way that patterned Christ's ministry. Christ first met the needs of the people. This might include restoring vision, helping the lame to walk, or curing leprosy. He did not judge. He did not have a condescending attitude. He served.

After He met their acute needs, He then began to teach them truth using parables. Along the way, He revealed the deceptions of the time. He introduced them to love and the path to ultimate healing. His approach was available to and understandable by everyone.

In the first part of the book, I've tried to introduce you to the problem. Remember, if you don't understand the problem, it's difficult to find the solution. David had a need when he was having a heart attack. After the acute need was met, I began to teach him.

The problem, as we've discovered, is stress—stress on our genetics, stress from the foods we eat, stress in our thoughts, basically anything we do that goes against the way we were designed. This activates chemistry, damaging the body and leading to symptoms and the need for acute care. Stress has been going on since the beginning, but it seems to be escalating in the times in which you and I live.

Now that we have a framework in regards to the problem, it is time to write about the solution.

I want to get something right out in the open. I suspect you know what is coming next, but I want to say it anyway. I believe in a God who created the world and the laws governing it. I believe in a God who has the power to heal and has infused His healing power deep within our own bodies. Finally, I believe God wants us all to be aware of and utilize the gifts He has provided so we can begin to overcome sickness of the mind, body, and spirit.

THE HEART OF HEALTH: AVOIDING DECEPTION

This may sound a bit strange coming from a man of science, but it is true. While some in my profession focus entirely on the achievements of technology, the amazing intellect of those who create the technology, and who—for want of a better word—seem to *worship* the science behind medicine and healing, I feel they are missing something important.

If I am having a heart attack, I definitely want a stent implanted in my coronary artery by a skillful physician. I'm going to be overjoyed that such science and technology are available, even though medications and medication errors can be a leading cause of death if misused. If I have a bacterial infection, I want an antibiotic. As I have said before, there's a place for modern medicine. Always has been. Always will be.

But I also have come to realize that disease does not just jump into our bodies. In more cases than not, we put it there. We are now beginning to understand the chemistry driving both health and disease, and as we continue to gain more understanding, many in the scientific community are beginning to appreciate the logic behind what the Creator did almost 6,000 years ago. As a matter of fact, I have come to the place in my own life where "Creator logic" trumps man's understanding every time. Even if I don't fathom why God did something, I know there must have been a good reason, and I find satisfaction in searching for the reason.

When it comes to how we are supposed to interact with God, He does not ask for blind faith. To paraphrase the words of a popular gospel song of a few years back, God never says, "I said it, and you believe it, and that should be good enough for you."

Our God is a logical, highly scientific being. He does not work in the shadows or keep His cards close to His chest. In one of the most thrilling texts in the Bible, the One who made us invites "Come now, let us reason together" (Isaiah 1:18). "I have nothing to hide," He seems to be saying. "I will tell you everything you want to know."

Then we read this incredible statement. "I will instruct you and teach you in the way you should go; I will counsel you and watch over you. Do not be like the horse or the mule, which have no understanding but must be controlled by bit and bridle or they will not come to you" (Psalm 32:8, 9). How many of us are being controlled by powers other than our own understanding? How many of us are bridled to the media, to the Internet, to some health fad that will soon be proven flawed or even dangerous?

I want you to consider trusting God in a way you have never trusted Him before. I want you to begin worshipping the God who created science instead of worshipping at the altar of human interpretation of that science. This is at the core of the solution.

Hands-on God

As I said earlier, years ago I read a book by Josh McDowell titled *More Than a Carpenter.* It provided fascinating examples of events predicted in the Bible that were fulfilled over the centuries. The book presented case after case in which archaeology proved the Bible's accuracy. This reinforced my belief in the God who not only created me, but also remained involved in the history leading up to my birth. This God is totally "hands-on." He was—and is— always ready to reason with anyone willing to listen to Him.

Would that be you? Are you ready to listen?

Something else I discovered about God. He cannot lie. It's not that He doesn't. He *can't*. He cannot even tell a "white" lie. He is all about truth. When He says something, it happens. Period.

As I was moving down this path during my college years at the University of Texas, I began recognizing that scientific and prophetic evidence were coming together to prove the truth in the Bible. And in this process of gathering evidence, I slowly but surely was also developing a relationship with God. Suddenly, God was not some distant power simply observing my progress through life. He became real to me—a force, a presence to whom I could turn when the questions got too big to bear.

This experience is what I want for my children. This is what I want for my patients. This is what I want for you.

The Secret Is the Search

The story is told of a physics professor whose specialty was energy and matter. Year after year, in his classroom at the university, he opened up to his students the great mysteries of the universe, teaching them how matter could be turned into energy, how energy could make matter, and how speed and time were interrelated. He proposed a theory to explain how God could be at all places at all times based on the manipulation of time and speed. Even though his class was challenging, there was a waiting list of students hoping for a place at his feet.

Open-minded students tended to do well. Status quo seekers—those who simply wanted to memorize a bunch of words or concepts—usually had problems in his class and struggled for a passing grade. Not surprisingly, the administration was constantly giving him grief about his methods, but the results reflected in the lives of many who took his class, and the deep love felt by the students for the man, served to produce strong arguments he was truly onto something valuable.

Near the end of one semester, the professor informed his students there would be a final physics test the following week. When the day arrived, those in the class sat expectantly, waiting to see what their instructor had in store for them. "Your final test for this class is a simple one," he announced. "I am going to divide you into teams and give each team the chance to assemble and run this small automobile." He pulled the covering off of a diminutive foreign car at the front of the class. "It's mostly assembled already and there is fuel in the tank. All you have to do is complete the assembly, start it, and drive it 10 feet."

Then the professor held up a block of paraffin and seven blank keys. "Oh, and you will have to create the key that starts the ignition. Good luck."

Each team was also handed a test booklet with these additional guidelines: 1. Read these instructions first: 2. Remember the big picture in figuring out how to make this car run successfully: 3. Start by inflating the tires: 4. Move on to the fuel and other systems next.

The students gathered in their teams and went over the challenge: blank keys, a block of paraffin, nearly assembled car, no questions to answer, no complex mathematical formulas to work, no calculus to use, no aerodynamics to ponder. Piece of cake!

The professor informed his students they would all make an A if they could get the car to start and drive it 10 feet.

The students attacked the problem with enthusiasm. Some immediately hooked up the fuel system. Some tried to make keys by etching grooves in the blanks provided. Still others checked the electrical system, making sure power was getting from the battery to the starter coil. One team even had the forethought to test the provided fuel, making sure it was the type the engine needed.

At the end of the first hour, the car still sat there unstarted and unmoving.

One student carefully watched the actions of the others, trying to fathom what the professor was attempting to teach with this unconventional test. He glanced over at the professor, who sat at his big desk watching the class thoughtfully. What was everyone missing? What were they not doing right?

That is when his eyes fell on the instruction booklets lying scattered about the room. No one was reading it. No one was following its carefully printed guidelines.

The student picked up his copy and started to reread the professor's words. *1. Read these instructions first.* Many had done that, but after reading them, they had simply headed off on their own paths, hoping their own knowledge would solve the problems. *2. Remember the big picture in figuring out how to make this car run successfully.* The student suddenly realized the "big picture" not only included the car; it included the instruction booklet as well. *3. Start by inflating the tires.* A quick glance at the automobile's tires revealed no one had done this. Why inflate the tires of a car that can't run?

The student walked over to the test car and began pumping air into rubber. As the fourth tire swelled to full inflation, he noticed something had been drawn on the sidewall—a finely detailed outline . . . of a key.

Wordlessly, the student carefully copied the outline onto the paraffin wax, created an indentation in the wax based on the outline, strolled over to a heat source, melted several of the blank keys in a pan, and then poured the molten liquid into the paraffin outline. When the newly cast key had cooled, he lifted it out, brushed away the imperfections, got into the car, started the engine, and drove across the room.

In our world, our minds are being influenced. More to the point, they are often being deceived. We think we know the answers, but we don't. God does, and He has provided those answers in a very obvious place—His Holy Word. He has not hidden them. He hasn't shut them away from our searching eyes. But He does require something of us. To discover how to "start" our journey back to optimum health and "drive" our lives to a satisfying end, we need to read—and follow—the simple guidelines He has provided.

You do not begin your journey back to health at your doctor's office. You do not search the Internet for answers to your most troubling questions. This can all come later. But first, you simply go to your bookshelf and retrieve the most sold but least read book this world has ever known. You sit down in a quiet place, open its pages, and begin to read. Because it is here that you will discover the key to ignite the change you've been longing to bring into your life.

As we continue the search for the solution, let's begin the journey together in the very first book of the Bible.

Vision of Things to Come

I wish I could have been there in the very beginning. Try to imagine the scene with me. We see earth's first couple, fresh from the mind and hand of God, surrounded by a garden teeming with life. It's day 7 of Creation week, the day God has set apart as earth's official rest day.

The Creator joins the happy pair by a bubbling brook and they admire the flowers and animals that make this new home such a pleasure. Then God turns to Adam and Eve and says, "Be fruitful and increase in number; fill the earth and subdue it. Rule over the fish of the sea and the birds of the air and over every living creature that moves on the ground" (Genesis 1:28). In other words, He is inviting the couple to care for His new creation; nurture the land and love the animals—an assignment they accept with great joy.

Then God says, "'I give you every seed-bearing plant on the face of the whole earth and every tree that has fruit with seed in it. They will be yours for food. And to all the beasts of the earth and all the birds of the air and all the creatures that move on the ground—everything that has the breath of life in it—I give every green plant for food.' And it was so. God saw all that he had made, and it was very good" (verses 29-31).

Right then and there, on the seventh day of Creation, surrounded by all that breathtaking beauty, God revealed something important to us all. His work of creation was complete. His great labor of love had ended. Everything Adam and Eve needed to live a happy, healthy life was right there in the garden with them. More to the point, God's "Health Plan"—a plan constructed from pure love, capable of holding the world and all creation in perfect harmony—was now in full effect, waiting to be enjoyed by every living thing. Nothing else was needed. In today's world, this is hard to imagine.

Here is what many of us fail to realize today. That loving Health Plan is *still* in effect—is *still* operating, is *still* the most powerful, concise, and effective way to build and maintain optimum health. It can still bring health and harmony to anyone's body, mind, and spirit.

In taking a careful look at the world as Adam and Eve experienced it and as God created it, we can gain incredible insights into how we are supposed to live, and how we can survive optimally in our own fast-paced, anything goes, if-it-feels-good-do-it world today. The laws God set in motion during those seven days of Creation are waiting to bring healing to our minds and bodies today—no matter how much we have abused those principles in the past.

I have seen those laws of love at work in my patients—bringing healing when all else seemed to fail, changing the chemistry, relieving stress placed on a system. Time and time again, the scientific community has proven God's way is the best way—that His health laws are more powerful than pharmaceuticals, medical devices, or high-tech procedures in dealing with and helping prevent chronic illnesses.

Most exciting of all, utilizing God's health laws is inexpensive and universal.

Would you like to know what those laws are? Would you like to discover what God had in mind for your body, your mind, and your relationship with your Creator? Let's spend some time digging into the story of Creation to discover those vital principles and learn how to apply them to our lives today.

Chapter 7

Day 1—From Darkness to Light

In the beginning God created the heavens and the earth. Now the earth was formless and empty, darkness was over the surface of the deep, and the Spirit of God was hovering over the waters. And God said, "Let there be light," and there was light. God saw that the light was good, and he separated the light from the darkness. God called the light "day" and the darkness he called "night." And there was evening, and there was morning—the first day (Genesis 1:1-5).

I t was now time to introduce David to the original plan for health: the Owner's Manual I had given him. This plan was perfect and given to this world at Creation. This plan was also designed with you and me in mind. Unfortunately, a host of deceptions that continue to this very day has sidetracked us. As we have moved away from this plan, stress has entered our bodies at every level. I needed to get David to understand the importance of the original design.

When the Creator began His work, He did not have a lot to work with. Genesis 1:1 reveals, "the earth was formless and empty, darkness was over the surface of the deep." Not exactly a choice vacation spot. But there is more. There was not any light. I am not talking about the absence of a sun or moon. I'm saying light could not even exist there.

How is that possible? Allow me to speculate. Have you ever heard of a black hole? Scientists are discovering more and more of these mysterious regions sprinkled throughout the known universe. Black holes are so dense, so packed with incredible power, so heavy with gravity, light cannot even exist within them. Some scientists suggest that the material that would soon become our world was floating around in the middle of a black hole when God began His transformations.

No one knows for sure how the Creator created, but the first thing He did was make light *possible* in our dark world. He spoke, and suddenly there was light (Genesis 1:3). The condition that had gripped our world in darkness was gone with a simple command from God. God provided the light.

Which leads me to this question: Are you living in a physical, mental, or spiritual "black hole"? Are you so imprisoned by destructive health habits, bitterness and shame, anger and lust, sadness and feelings of revenge that the light of God's love cannot even exist in your life? If so, the very first step, in God's Health Plan, is the same step taken on the first day of Creation. The Creator made light *possible*. That is exactly what He is waiting to do for you if you will just give Him access to the dark corners of your heart. He wants to be the light of your life, the solution to a dark, stress-filled world.

Let me give you an illustration of what I am talking about. A woman stands at the rain-splashed window of her home gazing out at a threatening storm. Her husband and children are an hour overdue from their outing. Thunder rattles the windows, lightning flashes, and the woman's heart trembles with fear. She has not eaten supper, she cannot relax, her head is throbbing with concern, and her stomach aches with worry.

Suddenly she sees the lights of the car in the driveway and the smiling, laughing faces of her children. Her husband waves apologetically as he guides the automobile into the garage.

In that instant, the woman discovers . . . she's hungry! Her heart returns to its normal rhythm. No more stomachache. No more pounding head. No more worry. Her family is safe, and she feels a great relief flooding her entire body. This is the way she is supposed to feel.

This is what happens when God's light of love enters a darkened life. We now experience how we were designed to feel. We become aware of destructive health habits needing to be set aside. When God's love illuminates a life, the transformation can begin.

Two-edged Sword

I must add this light of love is a two-edged sword because, many times, things long hidden become painfully obvious once the light is turned on, issues we cannot see in the darkness. Have you ever shined a flashlight under your bed? If you haven't, be prepared for a shock. You will find stuff under there you have not seen since Reagan was president. Light reveals much. It sometimes illuminates perhaps more than we'd prefer. But you have got to know what is making you sick before you can find healing. The light of truth helps us to see and open our eyes.

Once God has taken up residence in your heart, the light will be turned on. The original plan given at Creation started with light on day 1. When you receive this light, you will desire to activate His Health Plan in your life. It will be time to get to work, removing variables in your environment that could contribute to your physical, mental, or spiritual stress. Out go the unfit magazines and books, the violent DVDs, the toxic chemicals under the kitchen sink, the sugar- and salt-laden processed foods with little or no nutritional value, the Web sites filled with images that pollute the mind, the music promoting selfish thoughts and actions. With God's help you will work out the poisons in your life that have been slowly destroying you for years. The darkness is replaced by God's healing light.

Sometimes, what is needed most in our lives is simply the awareness of God's presence. My 9-year-old son, Jake, provided a wonderful example of this recently. One night he tiptoed into our bedroom, saying he had a scary dream. Next he snuggled up close to me, and that is where he remained until dawn. He did not say a word. He just needed the touch and presence of his father. His darkness—the darkness of 9-year-old boys who sometimes have scary dreams—was chased away by the love he felt from me, a love I was more than happy to share.

During our lives, we may experience "scary dreams." One might include a health challenge, even for those of us who do our best to follow God's Health Plan. Our overstressed bodies do eventually wear out. But we know where to find wonderful light, even when all else fails. We know of a power capable of bringing a world into being from utter and complete emptiness. We know of a love that shines a light into the darkest corners of our lives and is able to make something out of nothing.

On the first day of Creation, God demonstrated He was able to bring light into the darkest places. That is what He wants to do with each one of us today. He wants us to be aware of His constant presence.

Chapter 8

Day 2—Breathing Lessons

And God said, "Let there be an expanse between the waters to separate water from water." So God made the expanse and separated the water under the expanse from the water above it. And it was so. God called the expanse "sky." And there was evening, and there was morning—the second day" (Genesis 1:6-8).

Anyone who has ever taken an ocean voyage can imagine what the end result of day 2 of Creation week looked like. You see an endless expanse of ocean spreading out to the horizon. Above that, a blue sky, and hovering over it all float white, billowing clouds made up of . . . water—water separated from water with air in between.

So, how does this second day of Creation play into God's Health Plan for our lives? The answer is obvious, but all too often in the twenty-first century the fundamentals of life are overlooked in favor of the latest trends in technology. It makes perfect sense that after giving us light to take away darkness, God would give water and air, key ingredients for our survival and also key components needed for health and the treatment of disease. Without either, we would die. I explained to David, "When you had a heart attack and went to the emergency room, what did they do first? They hooked you up to oxygen and started an IV so they could give you fluids."

"No problem," I hear you say. "I breathe all the time. As for water, I make sure I don't go thirsty by drinking plenty of liquids."

There is just one problem. Sure, we breathe—we pull oxygen into our bodies. But, what else comes in with each of those breaths? And as for the liquids we consume each day, just how much of it is actually water?

THE HEART OF HEALTH: AVOIDING DECEPTION

Life and Breath

Breathing is a way to change our chemistry. Just try holding your breath for a period of time and you will notice some very definite changes taking place. When we breathe we introduce oxygen into our body. Holding your breath can lower your oxygen levels and raise your carbon dioxide levels. Breathing fast can lower the carbon dioxide levels. Breathing either too slow or too fast can affect the acid-base balance in the body. My point is breathing is important. God, as recorded in Genesis 2, "breathed into his [Adam's] nostrils the breath of life, and the man became a living being" (verse 7). Life and breath go together.

The effect of oxygen is profound. Our tissues need oxygen for survival. Ever wonder why you usually feel so good, so alive, while walking along a beach? The ocean is a veritable oxygen factory, releasing copious amounts of this precious element into the atmosphere from its submerged vegetation. We breathe in the oxygen-rich air and feel wonderful!

However, catching a good breath of air, which draws in the needed amount of oxygen, is getting a little more challenging these days. Stress can alter our breathing patterns. When our bodies are under stress, we breathe faster and shallower. This might be advantageous if we are in a fight for our lives—or our body is responding to some acute *and temporary* situation, but stressful breathing for extended periods of time is damaging. Long-term stress means long-term lack of optimal breathing.

Then there's sleep apnea.

Martin ventured into my office a few years ago. He easily weighed 450 pounds and stood only five feet eight inches tall. Unhappy about his health, he did not know where to begin to turn things around. Depression had set in as he struggled with diabetes, high blood pressure, fatigue, headaches, and a litany of joint pains. Martin could not walk across the room without getting short of breath and running his heart rate up to 140 beats a minute. Yes, life had turned into a struggle for this 39-year-old. He had never planned for this to happen, but one thing led to another and . . . you get the picture. His 15 prescription medications caused many side effects.

One of Martin's challenges was an ailment known as sleep apnea. This is a condition in which one does not get enough oxygen at night. Lack of oxygen means lack of sound sleep, which brings about lack of tissue renewal. The whole body becomes stressed. Martin had been stressed by this one third of his life. Can you imagine going underwater, holding your breath as long as possible, then coming up for a breath? This was what Martin was essentially doing eight hours a day. Sleep apnea alone could explain the high blood pressure, headaches, fatigue, and palpitations he was experiencing. Poor Martin.

I explained the acute treatment for sleep apnea—the sleep mask to force oxygen into his lungs, and possible surgery, if indicated, to help open a blocked airway. However, as you have discovered throughout this book, acute care usually only addresses symptoms and not necessarily the cause of those symptoms. I needed to offer more. My patient was searching for a new approach, a hint of hope, and the ability to love himself back to health.

Does this sound familiar? Isn't that what we all need when facing seemingly insurmountable health problems? We often ask ourselves, "Is traditional medicine the way to go? Is there something more? Where are the answers for which I am searching?"

Martin began with a common request. "Doctor Marcum, can't you just give me a pill to make me feel better?" I explained to him the easiest thing in the world for me to do would be to prescribe yet another medication—number 16 in his case. But this would not solve the underlying problem. We needed to go a step further. We needed to be honest. And I knew honesty had to be wrapped in love. I was not just dealing with a symptom. I was dealing with a living, breathing person. Truth was, Martin's problem was his weight and the behaviors leading to the weight.

I am ashamed to admit it, but money and selfishness greatly influence the treatment of disease these days. There are many people making money from the sick. The cigarette industry, the fast-food industry, the health insurance industry, hospitals, producers of medical supplies, the government, drug companies, and, yes, even physicians profit from people's suffering. The more people suffer, the more others profit. For instance, much more money is made from a bypass surgery or from taking prescription medications than is made from preventing a problem or dealing with the stress, which will cause problems down the road. Do not misunderstand me. I believe in and practice modern medicine. But there are often better solutions than a pill and a bill for every ill.

As I explained this to Martin, I could see him gaining interest and, more important, hope. He needed to lose weight. He needed to make some major changes in his lifestyle. He needed to return to God's Health Plan. I told him sometimes the best medicine is no more medicine. That's right. Sometimes the best way to heal a body is to get out of the way and let the incredible healing powers God gave do their own thing unencumbered by drugs. We enact the prescriptions given at Creation.

This may be hard for society to swallow when we spend one in six dollars of gross domestic product (GDP) on health care. But the truth is, chronic illness is not caused by a lack of pharmaceuticals. Breaking the divine laws of health is the real culprit. God created air for an important reason. Martin was robbing himself of this vital element by allowing himself to become obese. Obesity was causing an obstruction of his airway when he was in the prone position. Lose weight, breathe better, and healing sleep is restored. The answer to Martin's sleep apnea was not to be found in a bottle of pills. It was to be found at the dinner table.

My patient left my office with a renewed determination and a set of suggestions for curbing his appetite for unhealthy foods.

Relaxing Breaths

Breathing not only brings oxygen into the body; it can also help relax it. When you feel under stress, change your chemistry! Begin taking slow deep breaths through the nose. Hold for a few seconds and exhale. You will sense your body beginning to relax. This type of breathing is especially useful at night when you are preparing to rest, as this relaxes the body while enhancing oxygen delivery to the tissues.

A hundred years ago, lack of oxygen was not really much of an issue. Physical work such as plowing a field or building a barn provided that type of deep breathing automatically. Walking instead of driving offered the same benefit. But, as the world has changed, so have our breathing patterns. We need to get back to the basics of our chemistry, and nothing is more basic than breathing.

Right now, if you happen to be in a clean-air environment, I want you to take a few slow, deliberate deep breaths. Draw the air in through your nose. Hold for four or five seconds, and then blow it out completely through your mouth. Now, repeat. Then repeat again. See? Don't you feel more relaxed? The influx of oxygen just slowed your heart rate, lowered your blood pressure, and made your tissue very, very happy. No pill required.

The Challenge

Breathing in enough oxygen should not be a problem for many of us. But some may face a challenge or two in this area. More and more homes and offices are tightly sealed to save energy costs. The result is poor ventilation and the accumulation of indoor air pollutants. Formaldehyde, for example, seeps from certain wood products. Various fumes escape from carpets, copy machines, upholstery, and cleaning products. Carbon monoxide and nitrogen dioxide—two poisonous gases—rise unseen from gas, oil, or coal furnaces; ranges; fireplaces; and heaters. Mix in a good dose of dust, air mites, molds and fungi, ozone, lead, asbestos, pesticide residues, and a dash of radon gas and, well, suddenly the air we breathe takes on a rather sinister character. Yet how many warning labels do you see on synthetic household items or hanging over the door of your place of business? Remember, we were not designed to live indoors with this type of air. We were created to be outdoors breathing pure, unpolluted air.

In some areas, outside air may not be much of an improvement. Diesel fumes, factories spewing pollutants into the atmosphere, cars everywhere coughing out their by-products, and even your neighbor mowing his postage-stamp-size lawn with a 24-horsepower riding mower is not exactly helping the situation. Do you see warnings printed on the sides of trucks or fastened on the steering wheels of riding mowers?

What are some of the results of breathing pollutant-laden air? Burning eyes, sore throats, coughing, itching, headaches, sluggishness, nausea, dizziness, feelings of exhaustion, and depression—the very type of symptoms millions take to their doctors in order to get that "magic" and usually costly pill to address the problem.

Suddenly, enjoying the clean air brought into existence on the second day of Creation seems like an impossible dream. How can we take advantage of this powerful element of God's Health Plan for our lives?

Here are some suggestions. First, ban all smoking indoors and out. Even secondhand smoke contains hundreds of harmful chemicals.

Second, make sure your gas, oil, kerosene, and coal-burning heaters and appliances are well vented.

Third, keep air ducts and filters of heating and air-conditioning units well maintained. Make sure your chimneys are open and in good repair.

Finally—and this is so simple and important—keep fresh air coming into your home or office by opening a window. Even in the dead of winter, open a window just a crack to allow clean, fresh air access to your home or office. In some areas, you might want to make sure the window can't be opened any farther for safety's sake.

Breathe deeply of God's fresh air every day and keep a good supply of oxygen coursing through your body with regular exercise. Remember, God created the sky for a reason.

Water of Life

The second element of God's Health Plan that showed up on that second day of Creation was water. Not soda. Not milk. Not even fruit juice. Water!

I recently read a report from Loma Linda University. It had to do with this amazing liquid.

It is common knowledge that not drinking enough water has been linked to such ailments as constipation, kidney stones, overeating, and dry eyes, mouth, and skin. This new study, published in the *American Journal of Epidemiology*, showed that drinking high amounts of plain water is as important as exercise, diet, or not smoking in preventing coronary heart disease.

While that bit of information was surprising enough, what caught my eye was the word "plain" next to the word "water." According to the study, neither total fluid intake nor intake of other fluids combined showed this reduced risk. Coffee, soda, milk, and caffeinated drinks offered no significant heart benefits. In fact, these types of fluids draw water *from* the blood because they cannot be absorbed until their concentration is similar to that of the blood. *Plain* water, however, is absorbed immediately and quickly hydrates the system, thinning the blood and, thus, reducing the risk of clots that can lead to a heart attack.

The study concluded with these words: "Because drinking more plain water is a simple lifestyle change that anybody can do, this practice has the potential of saving tens of thousands of lives each year with minimal cost."

Listen to how Jesus, speaking to a woman at a well, labeled His presence in a life. "Whoever drinks the water I give him will never thirst. Indeed, the water I give him will become in him a spring of water welling up to eternal life" (John 4:14). His love does the same thing to a person's spiritual life as water does for his or her physical life. Jesus recognized the importance of water given on day 2 of Creation.

Divine Dilution

After reading the Loma Linda study, a dark thought crossed my mind concerning my own spiritual health. How often do I dilute God? How often do I accept the God my church portrays or the God of my favorite sermon CD or the God of the latest best seller as my Savior? How often do I add a little extra ingredient to my relationship with Him that actually accomplishes nothing to enhance His power in my life? All these things do is make God "taste" better in my mind or make Him "blend" more unobtrusively with my appetite for worldly deceptions.

I am determined to build my relationship with the "plain" God I find when I close my eyes in prayer or walk in the shaded solitude of a forest. As a matter of fact, if enough of you will join me, we will create our own "scientific" study that will end with these words: "Because worshipping the 'plain' God is a simple lifestyle change that anybody can do, this practice has the potential of saving tens of thousands of souls each year with minimal cost."

God's Health Plan includes *plain* water—not the "messed-with" liquid we find in colorful bottles and cans at the grocery store. It's not fruit juices, vegetable mixtures, or all-natural smoothies—healthy enough in their own right—that God created on that second day. He made water—plain and simple. Unfortunately, many of us bypass that "no-caloric wonder" on a regular basis.

It is common knowledge in the medical community that a vast majority of Americans are suffering from dehydration. In fact, it is estimated up to 70 percent of us do not hydrate ourselves adequately. It is not fun to walk in a hot desert. It causes the stress chemistry to be activated. Imagine, in a land where clean water is as close as your kitchen sink, we're robbing our bodies of one of the most important elements needed for a healthy life.

Water lubricates the body parts, flushes out impurities, protects us from diseases, and keeps us going when others fade. As a matter of fact, Africans have another name for this liquid that we should keep in mind. In their countries, water is simply called "life."

So, how much water should you drink? Here's a simple rule to follow. The average adult body loses around 10 to 12 cups of water a day through the skin, lungs, urine, and feces. A whole-foods, plant-based diet provides up to four cups of water, leaving us eight cups short. This should be added to our systems using plain, unmessed-with water filtered straight from the tap or well. Another suggestion is take your body weight and divide in two. This is approximately how many ounces of water are needed each day for a healthy person.

Want a great start for your day? Drink a glass of room-temperature water right after you get up, then again in midmorning. Want to keep going and going and going? Enjoy another glass of water in midafternoon and again in early evening. And, at all times, follow this simple rule: If you're thirsty, drink *water*.

The real reason we are becoming more and more sick as a society is we are losing sight of what God had in mind for keeping us healthy when He created us. Water and air were created on day 2 for an important reason. We have a tendency to turn our eyes away from His simple yet powerful truths given at the beginning. We tend to focus our attention on science and technology to heal our ills. It is so important that we return to the basics.

As I finished, David agreed that before today he didn't even think about water and air as treatments that were as important as his prescriptions. He was becoming more eager to learn. He was discovering truth. He began to hear God's voice speaking. He could hardly wait for day 3.

Chapter 9

Day 3—Health on Solid Ground

And God said, "Let the water under the sky be gathered to one place, and let dry ground appear." And it was so. God called the dry ground "land," and the gathered waters he called "seas." And God saw that it was good.

Then God said, "Let the land produce vegetation: seed-bearing plants and trees on the land that bear fruit with seed in it, according to their various kinds." And it was so. . . . And there was evening, and there was morning—the third day (Genesis 1:9-13).

What if I told you scientists had unearthed something that would greatly lower or, in some cases, completely remove your risk of cancer, heart disease, and diabetes. Interested? Well, the amazing breakthrough is available today—not at the drugstore, but at your local grocery store; note I said *grocery* store.

I recently heard a story from an international development and relief agency. Seems that in Mongolia, winters had been especially severe—so severe in fact many of the animals the people depended on for food died. The good folk at the agency knew that if something was not done right away, many Mongolians would perish from starvation. Their food source was dying in the cold.

So they rolled up their sleeves and got to work, teaching people how to grow vegetable gardens using weather-resistant seeds, proper irrigation, and nonchemical fertilizers. Soon, neat, green rows of growing vegetables could be seen in garden plots large and small throughout the country. Little by little the diet of thousands of Mongolians changed from being *animal*-based to being *plant*-based. They now had vegetables to eat and were not solely dependent on animals.

As hoped, starvation was averted. The people who had gardens survived very well and were even able to help their neighbors stay alive. After the agency showed them how to build economical storage buildings, communities began enjoying sufficient supplies of garden-grown food year-round.

But, that is not the end of the story. When representatives checked back with those who had adopted the new plant-based diet, they learned something interesting. Children who ate their veggies instead of meat suffered from fewer colds and other illnesses. Adults enjoyed more energy and health, bypassing many of the sicknesses sweeping the country. Not only were they alive; they were alive *and well*. All they had done was alter their diet to be plant-based.

This really should not surprise us. After all, what those Mongolians had done was, unknowingly, adopt a powerful component of God's Health Plan— a plan He created right along with the rest of this earth.

At the end of the third day of Creation week, the Creator left behind, not a world "formless and empty," as it was before. No, He left a world covered with land, sea, vegetation, and sky. In other words, God had created a farm! One problem. Any schoolchild knows plants need more than air and water to grow. They need something else. They need the sun.

That is why the very next day, God said, "'Let there be lights in the expanse of the sky to separate the day from the night. . . .' God made two great lights— the greater light to govern the day and the lesser light to govern the night" (Genesis 1:14-16).

On that fourth day, this world fairly exploded with plant life after the sun appeared. Have you ever seen those time-lapse movies of flowers opening up or vines growing along stone walls? In those amazing film clips, days and weeks are compressed into mere seconds. That is what it may have looked like when the plants created on day 3 found themselves staring up at day 4's sun. It must have been an awesome sight! We will explore the powerful health-building properties of the sun in our next chapter.

But, just for a moment, let's move to the end of Creation week when God is standing with Adam and Eve in their new garden home. The Creator's arm sweeps over the verdant growth surrounding them, indicating the fruit-heavy trees and produce-laden plants. With a satisfied smile, He turns to the happy couple. "I give you every seed-bearing plant on the face of the whole earth," He tells them in verse 29, "and every tree that has fruit with seed in it. They will be yours for food." This was the original diet for which our bodies were designed.

Which brings us back to the Mongolians—when they changed their diet more toward the foods God intended for humans to eat, their health improved. Their minds became clearer; their energy levels increased. No, we should not be surprised. Instead, we should try to return to that original plan. Just as light, water, and air are vital treatments for the body, so is the food we eat. I was now teaching David about another biblical truth.

Why Plants?

So, what is so special about fruits and vegetables? What do they have that animal products—foods made from animals—do not have? Actually, the more relevant question to ask is what do fruits and vegetables *not* have that animal-based products contain?

In his comprehensive report to the nation entitled *Nutrition and Health*, Surgeon General Dr. C. Everett Koop stated that the Western diet was a major contributor to heart disease, cancer, and stroke. He confirmed saturated fat and cholesterol found in abundance in animal protein of all kinds were the main culprits. He pointed out that these foods were usually eaten at the expense of complex-carbohydrate-rich selections such as whole grains, legumes, and vegetables.

In his book *Health Power* epidemiologist Dr. Hans Diehl states, "The risk for cancer of the prostate, breast, and colon is three to four times higher for people who consume meat, eggs, and dairy products on a daily basis when compared to those who eat them sparingly or not at all. In addition, vegetarian women have stronger bones and fewer fractures, and they lose less bone as they age."

To underscore his point, Diehl, the founder/director of CHIP (Coronary Health Improvement Project), adds research centered on long-lived vegetarians such as the Hunzas, who are healthy and active into advanced age, contrasts sharply with the short life span and increased disease rates of traditional Eskimos, who depend largely on what they catch in the sea or hunt on the frozen tundra.

Health studies and statistics are one thing. But, what do your eyes tell you when you walk through any mall in America or take part in any social gathering? Do we look healthy to you? Why are drugstore shelves lined with increasingly powerful head and stomachache medications? Why are obesity and diabetes rates soaring? Why are teenagers experiencing health problems that just a few years ago stalked only the elderly? The answer, to a large degree, is explained by diet. We are eating the wrong foods at the wrong times in the wrong amounts. And we are paying a terrible price for doing so.

God's Health Plan was complete at the end of Creation week. Adam and Eve needed nothing else—no wonder drugs, no pills or powders, no dietary supplements, no carbonated beverages, no fat-filled fast foods, no dairy products, no meat dishes, no heavily-refined foods in convenient take-home packaging. All they needed was right there before them in the garden. We as a world need to pay attention to this.

Modern Messages

Dr. T. Colin Campbell in his groundbreaking book *The China Study* took a balanced, unbiased, scientific look at the world's food sources and concluded a plant-based diet is the best way to go. Here's how he summed up his many years of study and research in the field of nutrition and health:

> "Almost all of us in the United States will die of diseases of affluence. In our China Study, we saw that nutrition has a very strong effect on these diseases. Plant-based foods are linked to lower blood cholesterol; animal-based foods are linked to higher blood cholesterol. Animal-based foods are linked to higher breast cancer rates; plant-based foods are linked to lower rates. Fiber and antioxidants from plants are linked to a lower risk of cancers of the digestive tract. Plant-based diets and active lifestyles result in a healthy weight, yet permit people to become big and strong. . . . From the labs of Virginia Tech and Cornell University to the far reaches of China, it seemed science was painting a clear, consistent picture: we can minimize our risk of contracting deadly diseases just by eating the right food" (p. 105).

Why don't we hear more about this? The answer is heartbreakingly sad. It is about the money. The media—and the advertisers who support the media—want to control our thoughts and buying tendencies. And, as I have said before, there is more money to be made by making and keeping us sick than by helping us get well. I am not surprised by Dr. Campbell's conclusion based on his decades of research. After all, the diet he found to be the healthiest was the very diet God placed before Adam and Eve 6,000 years ago in Eden: fruits, vegetables, nuts, grains, and plain water. No diet could be better. The scientific proof is there.

Even in the book of Daniel, we see this point driven home. This point was made for a reason. When offered the "affluent" diet of the king—a diet rich in animal protein and refined foods, which the poor people in the kingdom could not afford—Daniel and his friends proposed a test. Their story is found in Daniel, chapter 1. Let's begin with verse 8: "But Daniel resolved not to defile himself with the royal food and wine, and he asked the chief official for permission not to defile himself this way. Now God had caused the official to show favor and sympathy to Daniel, but the official told Daniel, 'I am afraid of my lord the king, who has assigned your food and drink. Why should he see you looking worse than the other young men your age? The king would then have my head because of you.'"

Does this sound familiar? "You need animal protein to grow big and strong!" advertisers shout from television sets and magazine pages. "Real men eat beef" and "Milk builds strong bones." We see beer manufacturers sponsoring sporting events, and the tobacco industry wants us to believe dumping more than 200 poisons into our lungs is "cool." But Daniel had a very different vision—one based not on the media, but on his Maker. He was acquainted with the Creation plan. Someone had taken the time to teach him. Daniel and his friends did not want the consequences, the bad chemistry, that would come with the king's food. Verse 11: "Daniel then said to the guard whom the chief official had appointed over Daniel, Hananiah, Mishael and Azariah, 'Please test your servants for ten days: Give us nothing but vegetables to eat and water to drink. Then compare our appearance with that of the young men who eat the royal food, and treat your servants in accordance with what you see.' So he agreed to this and tested them for ten days."

There was much at stake here, to say nothing of the chief official's head! These young men were willing to stand up for what they knew to be true even if by doing this they would be put at risk. So, how did his ancient health study play out? We find the results stated in verses 15-20: "At the end of the ten days they looked healthier and better nourished than any of the young men who ate the royal food. So the guard took away their choice food and the wine they were to drink and gave them vegetables instead. . . . At the end of the time set by the king to bring them in, the chief official presented them to Nebuchadnezzar. The king talked with them, and he found none equal to Daniel, Hananiah, Mishael and Azariah; so they entered the king's service. In every matter of wisdom and understanding about which the king questioned them, he found them ten times better than all the magicians and enchanters in his whole kingdom."

I don't know about you, but I think there's a definite message here for our public education system. Want smart kids? Feed them the right foods!

Acute Care

Modern medicine is great for acute care. Break a leg? We're there. Fighting an infectious disease? We're ready. Suffered a serious injury? Bring it on. But, we're not all that effective in dealing with the results of too many toxins, a sparseness of nutrients in many acres of overworked soil, and massive amounts of chemicals in our food, water, and air. Just as in Daniel's time, some of us cannot even think the way we should. The solution—as it was then—is to boost our intake of needed nutrients by selecting organic foods, detoxifying our bodies, and getting back to the Creator's original Health Plan.

Keep in mind that even "good foods" can be detrimental when loaded down with chemicals used to color, flavor, and preserve them. Read the labels. If you cannot pronounce an ingredient, you probably cannot digest it, either. Such additives and "enhancers" can create chronic stress on the system. We are now hearing about chemicals being leached from food storage containers and eventually entering our bodies. Chemicals from plastic, including bisphenol A, can stimulate our hormonal system sending signals that can cause damage to the body. Foreign estrogens called xenoestrogens do not belong in our body and can be very destructive to young people as they grow and develop, especially individuals with susceptible DNA.

Xenoestrogens have been found in plastics, pesticides, cosmetics, cleaners, and a host of other products. We wonder why we are seeing lower fertility rates, more prostate cancer, more birth defects, autism, and other conditions not seen before to this degree in our society. One hundred years ago, we just did not see these problems. What could be a possible cause?

Reports in the *Journal of the American Medical Association* (JAMA

2008:300[11]:1303-1310) have linked these chemicals with increased risk of cardiovascular disease, diabetes, and liver abnormalities. Recently a chemical called phthalates, which is also found in plastics, has been shown to damage the reproductive system and linked to cancer. Just think. In 2008 6 billion pounds of bisphenol A were produced.

Thanks to the information age, knowledge, as well as deception, gets around fast. But there is another problem facing those who are trying to follow God's original diet recommendations.

Mutant Munchies

Genetically modified foods are everywhere in our food supply. What are these? Genetic material with desired characteristics from a different species is inserted into the DNA of a plant or animal. For instance, genetic material is inserted in corn or cotton, which can enable it to make its own pesticide. Such a process is increasingly occurring in our food supply, and we do not really understand the long-term implications.

Toxic and allergic reactions have already been documented. Not only is genetic modification occurring in our food supply, but also this technology is being used in vaccines and drugs. Only common sense indicates there is a very good chance this will put stress on our bodies and affect our health. "But don't worry," says the medical profession, "we probably have a medication to mask the symptoms for a while. There is no data indicating danger." Well, what about common sense? What about the original plan? Is there data for this?

Just to put this into perspective and provide a tiny peek into the profits waiting to be made by the drug companies and health-care facilities, here are a few of the diseases and symptoms associated with chronic stress on our system: headaches, depression, anxiety, insomnia, Alzheimer's disease, panic disorders, eating disorders, obesity and subsequent health problems, diabetes, palpitations and abnormal heart rhythms, heart attacks, hypertension, infections because of weak immune systems, osteoporosis, ulcers, sexual dysfunction, acid reflux, irritable bowel syndrome, fibromyalgia, acne, psoriasis, eczema, shingles, arthritis, multiple sclerosis, lupus, chronic muscle and joint pain, and memory loss. I even probably missed a few. Are you beginning to see the broader picture here? Day 3's message is important to us all.

Mrs. Brown's Biscuits

Mrs. Brown is known for her great Southern biscuits. I have tasted them, and they are delicious! She is now 58 and grew up, like many of us, eating sugarcoated cereal in the morning, fast food at lunch during her work break, and then a large meal at night—sometimes topped off with a bowl of ice cream. Usually after eating, she watches television or surfs the Internet until bedtime.

I saw her in the office a few months ago. Her main complaint was a feeling of fatigue and constantly going to the bathroom. These symptoms were the tip of the iceberg. Testing revealed diabetes, high cholesterol, and hypertension. Most of these problems could be attributed to nutrition.

"You are what you eat" is a saying that has been passed down through the years. There is a lot of truth in the statement. Many, especially those in the fast-paced industrialized and highly technologic societies, have similar diets to Mrs. Brown's. We are approaching danger and are not even aware of it. Our culture promotes fast food, frozen food, salty food, fried food, high-caloric food, processed food, and too much food. This type of promotion is causing incredible amounts of suffering. Yes, this might be the more convenient way to eat, but it is totally messing up our chemistry and putting enormous stress on our system. We are being deceived into thinking we must follow the status quo and eat like we always have, the way we have been taught, or what we see in advertising. We must follow the leader and eat like everyone else. Where is that getting you? Where did that get David? What is happening to the world right in front of our eyes? What does the evidence say?

I, like most of you, have struggled with nutrition. I have fought against cultural pressure and the neuropathways of bad habits. It is a subject barely touched on in medical schools. Most hospitals fail to emphasize nutrition as treatment. And to further stir the waters, there seems to be a new nutrition or diet book published every week. Many are overwhelmed and confused by the wide variety of voices shouting out their messages. I wanted to give David, and I want to give to you, the reader, something simple and filled with commonsense logic based on day 3 of Creation. I also want to meet you where you are and give doable suggestions, recognizing sometimes change is slow.

Two important themes seem to remain consistent: 1. You are what you eat, and 2. Eating is a habit. There is much truth to these themes.

When I first started practicing medicine many years ago, I was very idealistic and encouraged my patients to eat perfectly. I remember one old-timer who looked over at me from his perch on the examination table. "Doc," he said, "I'd rather die than give up my fried 'taters."

Through the years, I have tried to develop a more realistic, commonsense approach to nutrition. I try to teach my patients what God designed us to eat while recognizing eating habits developed in childhood make up a large part of our persona.

This entire book has focused on biblical teachings: getting back to the original Owner's Manual outlined in Eden. I ask my patients, "What does God teach us about nutrition?" Then I refer them back to the often-overlooked verse in Genesis putting nutritional questions to rest. God, speaking to Adam and Eve, said, "See, I have given you every herb that yields seed which is on the face of all the earth, and every tree whose fruit yields seed; to you it shall be for food" (Genesis 1:29, NKJV).

Fuel

The story is told of a man who bought a brand-new car and proudly drove it home from the dealer's. But in just a few weeks, his pride and joy began to develop problems. It backfired constantly, smoked terribly, and was hard to start. The engine knocked continually and hardly developed any power to climb the smallest hill.

In a huff, the man jerked and backfired his way to the dealer, where he demanded his money back. "You sold me a lemon!" he said angrily.

The dealer walked around the car and peered under the hood at the overheated engine. "I don't understand," he said. "People love this particular model." Turning to the irate customer, he asked, "You are keeping oil and gasoline in it, aren't you?"

The man lifted his chin. "I put the best diesel fuel in it each and every week."

Opening the car's owner's manual, the dealer pointed to a notation on page 1. "Sir," he said, "this car was designed to run on regular, unleaded fuel, not diesel. That's what was causing *all* the problems. You were putting the wrong fuel into the tank."

Which begs the question, "What fuel are we putting into our bodies?" Our Owner's Manual, written by our Designer, has made it more than clear we are made to run on certain foods. He pointed them out, one by one, to Adam and

Eve. He makes them available to us today in our grocery store. Even science is showing the value of a plant-based diet consisting of fresh fruits, vegetables, nuts, and grains. The antioxidants and phytochemicals contained in these "fuels" promote health, fight inflammation, and give us boundless energy, while the diets high in fat—especially the trans-saturated fats found in most fast foods, damage our sometimes delicate systems.

The animals people eat are another major issue. The animals have their own set of health problems. To get them to market faster, chemicals are given to stimulate growth at an accelerated rate. These health problems and powerful chemicals are passed on to us when we eat their flesh or drink their milk. To put it simply, it is the wrong fuel, and can cause a cascade of problems within our bodies.

Shopping Trip

I am not much of a shopper. My wife, Sonya, will attest to that. I am also not too crazy about lugging bulging bags between specialty shops and superstores. But there is one type of shopping I can tolerate—*grocery* shopping. Just give me a list of foods the Marcum household needs and turn me loose!

When I shop, I like to head straight for the produce section of our favorite grocery store. Then I pause while imagining Adam and Eve standing in their garden looking over many of the same types of fruits, vegetables, grains, nuts, and legumes that I see. What a rainbow of colors meets my eye as I pick out my favorite fruits, dig through the display of vegetables, load up my cart with dried beans for the slow-cooker, choose the freshest whole-grain breads and cereals, and gather enough soy or rice milk to see us through the coming week. I have even learned to look for foods that are not genetically modified and are organic, thanks to my health-conscious wife. I now study labels and try to choose foods without all those long-worded chemicals in them. The less processing the better. Then I stand in line at the checkout counter as those around me study my collection with a touch of knowing in their eyes.

The Whole Truth

What is the best way to eat and how do I choose the foods highlighted in God's Health Plan? One word: *whole.* That means there is nothing missing. Everything that is supposed to be included is. The benefits are far-reaching. Diabetics, for instance, have for many years been instructed to stay away from sugars. Fruit juices are a no-no. But studies are revealing that if a diabetic eats the *whole* fruit—complete with fiber—his or her body responds more slowly and evenly to the natural sugars it contains and less damage is done.

God, in His infinite wisdom, created the foods that grow in the ground or hang from the trees in such a way we receive their full load of nutrition only when we eat them whole. All those powerful, cancer-fighting antioxidants, minerals, vitamins, and other healing nutrients find their way into our bodies via the fiber, juices, and protective coverings of those foods. *Whole* grains. *Whole* fruits. *Whole* vegetables, food as God intended.

When we start isolating the elements in foods and eating them far removed from their original form, we weaken their potential. That is what "refining" does—it separates elements into individual products. Sugarcane becomes table sugar, whole-wheat flour ends up as white flour, fruits get squeezed into fruit juices. The lowly potato is best served with its skin, even when mashed.

Healthy Love

Before we leave this amazing day of Creation, I want to share a thought with you. As we are discovering in the chapters of this book, building and maintaining optimum health takes more than making good food choices. It is also about the way we live, and what lives in our hearts. So many times I hear people dwelling only on the food aspect. Eat this. Don't eat that. Now, don't get me wrong; food is very important to health, but it is not the only component. I have even experienced some people getting angry, judgmental, or even depressed over their diet. These emotions are probably more dangerous than the unhealthy food they're telling everyone to avoid.

A sound body requires healthy thoughts, commonsense exercise, focused worship, and a thankful, loving heart. The Holy Spirit—if we will allow Him access to our minds—will lovingly lead us to physical health at the correct speed and through avenues we can trust. When we come to God with our shortcomings, He will give us the power to build and maintain optimum spiritual health as well. He does not want us to get down on others, or ourselves. God realizes what we have been through in life and it's about a journey, a relationship. Change sometimes must come slowly. I hope the Holy Spirit is touching you through this book.

When I see a person being judgmental or overreacting about any one aspect of their personal health plan, I am concerned. Please, do not make healthy habits a god. Do not worship at the throne of food, exercise, perfect lab numbers, ideal weight, or other health details. Worship the God who created you, and reflect His loving nature to those with whom you come in contact.

God has made it possible for all—even hungry Mongolians—to enjoy the health benefits and resultant good chemistry of eating the diet originally designed for our bodies. Now, that is a prescription I definitely want to fill.

Getting Real

Since the stress of eating foods devoid of nutritional value and high in saturated fats, salt, and sugar is such a big part of disease, I would like to take a few moments to offer a practical eating plan. It has been proven time and time again that if people make small, incremental changes in diet, three things happen: they start to feel better, they save money, and they enjoy more control over their health.

If you happen to be a runner, you will know exactly what I am talking about. You start out your run tired from the day's work, depressed over that argument with your spouse, and feeling "not so good." But a funny thing happens around block three. Something begins to change in your psyche. You find yourself strangely energized, even though you are expending energy. Your subconscious kicks in with a few suggestions on how to reconnect with the one you love, and you begin to feel better. The more you run, the more you want to run because it feels so good. You are experiencing a cascade of chemical changes in your body—changes that revive your mind, body, and spirit.

That is exactly what it's like when you begin making slow but steady nutritional adjustments. The "commonsense light" begins to illuminate in your awakening brain. Suddenly, you sense the danger in eating fatty foods as your doctor has warned concerning the fat that can build up in your arteries. If you are overweight, it begins to really sink in that you should eat less calories. If high blood pressure is a problem, you are suddenly shocked at the sodium numbers shouting at you from food labels. Like disease, health is self-perpetuating. There is no middle ground. Your lifestyle is either heading you for the hospital or for a happy retirement.

Eat Smart

So, how do you eat smart? Consider these suggestions that can save not only your heart, but your life. These suggestions might seem simplistic, but I have seen them work in my patients.

If you eat French fries every day, you might start by eating them only once a week, and then, maybe, just on special occasions like a birthday. If you eat greasy hamburgers every day at lunch, you might want to start by choosing a garden-burger-type meatless meal every other day, and toss in a salad with a little fat-free dressing on the side.

Hooked on colas? Substitute with a sweet, tangy fruit juice 50 percent of the time or—best of all—learn to enjoy the simple taste of water.

Gotta have morning coffee with its dangerous load of caffeine? Become more sophisticated and start enjoying hot herbal teas instead. Just try not to look too smug when your coworkers see you drinking it.

Once you begin making these small changes, your body chemistry will begin to improve and you will find yourself willing—dare I say eager—to make more changes because you feel much better.

When you eat can be just as important as what you eat. Many of my patients work all day, come home, eat a big meal comprised mostly of highly processed foods, flop down on the couch, watch television, and then finish out the evening with a bowl of ice cream. I do not mean to gross you out, but when we fill our stomachs with food—any food—late in the evening, then go to bed, the load of nutrients and "other stuff" kinda just sits there all night long. Not much digestion takes place while we sleep. It doesn't take much imagination to visualize what happens to organic material when it is stored for seven hours in a warm, moist place. Then, when we get up in the morning, we wonder why we feel so lousy, have absolutely no appetite, and our breath smells like the family cat crawled into the dirty clothes hamper and died.

I recommend you eat a much smaller meal as early in the evening as possible. Then you might want to head out for a short walk in the fresh air and burn off some of those calories.

Some people are able to make all the dietary changes I mentioned above at one time and are happy about the changes. They are probably in the minority. In creating a treatment plan based on good nutrition, I try to individualize the plan, remembering happiness is important, too. The "I'm going to change my lifestyle" mentality must place its focus on what you *can* do, not what you

THE HEART OF HEALTH: AVOIDING DECEPTION

can't. I *can* eat healthier food. I *can* live longer. I *can* cut my doctor bills. I *can* have more energy. I *can* bypass most of the disease plaguing modern society. I am not giving up food; I am simply changing my menu. In the great salad bar of life, I am choosing to load my plate with food God created especially for my body.

Practical Suggestions

This is not a nutrition book, but I do want to offer some more practical suggestions to improve your nutritional intake. I'll give it to you straight; what I've seen works best in my patients:

1. Eat a balanced diet with lots of fresh fruits, vegetables, nuts, whole grains, legumes, and seeds. This would include soy, rice, beans, and whole-grain pastas. Fad diets can be harmful.

2. Drink more water and avoid soft drinks. Stay away from anything that contains high fructose corn syrup. U.S. consumption of high fructose corn syrup went up 1000 percent between 1970 and 1990, according to a 2004 edition of *The American Journal of Clinical Nutrition*.

3. Avoid foods with a high-fat content: basically fried foods, meats, French fries, cheese, eggs, margarine and butter, ice cream, doughnuts, cookies, gravy, potato chips, and so on. These are high in trans-saturated fats, which cause all sorts of stress and chemical problems in the body.

4. Sparingly use monounsaturated fats such as olive oil and canola oil. You might learn how to leave them out completely. The body does not process such fats. It stores them. I do not have to tell you where.

5. Reduce salt intake by diminishing your use of table salt and processed foods. Remember, too much salt can increase blood pressure, which can lead to cardiovascular disease, kidney disease, osteoporosis, and kidney stones. In fact, half the people on dialysis are there because of high blood pressure.

6. Avoid eating *only* for pleasure. Eat when you are hungry; stop when you are full. Eat smaller portions slowly. By the way, foods high in fiber (plant-based foods) send a clear "I'm full" signal to the brain, which switches off the hunger sensation at just the right moment. Non fiber foods (animal products and highly processed foods) do not—something to think about.

7. Eat most of your calories in the morning. Not hungry when you get up? Simply eat a smaller supper and nothing after 6:00 p.m. When morning comes, food looks mighty good!

8. Become a vegetarian. Even most animals are vegetarians. When you eat meat, you are getting your calories secondhand. In addition, the diseases the animals might have and the steroids to promote growth and chemicals added to the animal's foods are passed on to you. Animal products are also absolutely loaded with fat. "But I'll just eat fish or only organic animal products," many patients say. While this is certainly a step in the right direction, meat protein is meat protein. Less is better. None is best.

9. Avoid the chemical additives found in most processed foods by avoiding processed foods. Here's a simple rule. Look for packaged foods with the fewest ingredients. Again, if you cannot pronounce an ingredient, you probably cannot digest it.

10. Eliminate caffeine and alcohol from your diet. These are two powerful toxins that do much more harm than good.

11. Be careful with supplements and herbs. Take the time to learn about them from a reliable source. Some herbs interfere with cardiac medications. It is always best to get your nutritional needs from whole foods—foods as grown.

12. Eat plenty of antioxidants. These amazing micronutrients have the incredible ability to fight the development and spread of cancer cells. Where do we find these antioxidants? They are found in plant-based foods such as fruits and legumes.

13. Find foods with omega-3, -6, -9 fatty acids—the healthy fats. Again, plant foods—almonds, walnuts, flaxseed. Grind flaxseeds before adding them to your diet.

I hope you are not overwhelmed after reading the list. Instead, I hope you are encouraged. There *is* hope for you and your family. There *is* a plan you can follow to bypass the bypass, to reduce the risk of contracting cancer, to shield yourself from the diseases filling doctors' offices and hospital beds.

Choose one or two items from the list and try to follow the suggestion for a month. It takes about a month to develop a habit. If you do this, I guarantee you will feel better. Once you get in the habit, pick another item from the list and work on it as well. As you feel better and more alive, the changes will become easier. Don't beat yourself up if you slip every now and then. Remember, it's a journey. You are in charge of your choices. When it comes to lifestyle diseases, you decide how sick you want to be.

THE HEART OF HEALTH: AVOIDING DECEPTION

Junk Money

The world wants you to eat poorly. There is a lot of money to be made when you eat "junk." There are deceptions at every turn. But, eating the right foods can change your chemistry and act just like medicines without the terrible side effects. Eating nutritionally devalued foods, however, can cause stress and can be compared to slow poison.

Many of our modern-day medications are derived from plants. There are actually entrepreneurs who search the world for powerful chemicals in plants and foods that help our bodies. Then, they isolate these chemicals and try to market them to us as the latest and greatest miracle cure, which can be ours for $19.95 plus tax and shipping. One problem. Isolating nutrients from their source removes them from the "delivery mechanism" God created for that nutrient. In isolation, sometimes these nutrients can become impotent.

Our friend Dr. Colin Campbell, in his book *The China Study,* calls this type of endeavor "scientific reductionism." Here's what he says: "As long as scientists study highly isolated chemicals and food components, and take the information out of context to make sweeping assumptions about complex diet and disease relationships, confusion will result. Misleading news headlines about this or that food chemical and this or that disease will be the norm."

Then Dr. Campbell concludes: "Scientific investigations of the effects of single nutrients on complex diseases have little or no meaning when the main dietary effect is due to the consumption of an extraordinary collection of nutrients and other substances found in whole foods."

Let me give you one example. Resveratrol is a phytochemical found in the skin of red grapes and other plants such as berries, plums, and peanuts. This chemical increases the activity of some sirtuin enzymes thought to be involved in the regulation of aging. Dietary supplements containing resveratrol are now being widely promoted as antioxidants that can slow or prevent age-related illnesses.

Wow! Pop a pill and slow aging and disease. But, guess what? Studies have shown caloric restriction (eating less) also increases sirtuin activity and a caloric restricted diet delayed the onset of age-related diseases and extended the life spans of primates in the lab.

So why would anyone want to shell out big bucks to buy an isolated part of certain foods when simply going to the grocery store and buying a nice bag of tasty red grapes, berries, plums, and nuts does exactly the same things without having to enroll yourself in a worldwide scientific study of what happens to the human body when it is introduced to an isolated nutrient from a whole food? Why not just eat the chemical as God gave it to us in nature?

I have an uneasy feeling that as time goes by we will begin hearing rumors of where that particular study is taking us.

But, are you hearing about studies that show the amazing health benefits of eating grapes, berries, plums, and nuts? No. Why? They are not moneymakers.

Before I end this section, let me give you some examples of foods with proven—under the marketing radar—chemical benefits. Pomegranate juice and soy milk can lower prostate specific antigen, i.e., PSA. Alzheimer's disease can be helped by the antioxidants found in blueberries, strawberries, and grapes. (These same antioxidants can also lower cholesterol and blood pressure.)

Turmeric and the vitamin D triggered in the body by sunlight can help fight breast cancer. Alpha omega fatty acids found in walnuts, almonds, flaxseed, and spinach can ease depression, lower cholesterol, and help nerve function.

Kelp can assist the thyroid. Oatmeal—or anything with fiber, such as almonds and walnuts, soy, and garlic—can lower cholesterol, thus decreasing the risk of cardiovascular disease. The benefits of beans, artichokes, chestnuts, carrots, onions, honey, pineapple, and almost any whole plant-based food you can think of now has the science to prove its chemical benefit. The list goes on and on as we learn more about the value of the chemicals God placed in the food He gave us to eat.

Indeed, the very food God gave us at the beginning can be treatment for the disease states we have inherited and acquired. But are we rushing to the produce section of our grocery stores so we can fight these diseases? No. We are forming lines at the drugstore, hoping the latest technological cure will keep us alive to see another day.

Why don't we hear God's Health Plan being shouted from the hilltops and televised with our favorite police drama? Where are the infomercials? Because God's not an entrepreneur. He is simply a loving Savior who makes good health available to anyone who can chew and swallow.

Our society puts those who murder behind bars. Yet dangerous foods literally killing us are promoted and not condemned. I just don't get it.

Don't be deceived. Do not make good nutrition harder than it needs to be. Use common sense. God will never be proven wrong by science because He created science. When making future food choices, pray for help. Whisper the words of the apostle Paul found in Philippians 4:13: "I can do everything through Him who gives me strength."

We have covered quite a bit in looking at day 3 of Creation. This information gave David a new appreciation for the food he eats. He now realizes the basic principles of nutrition were given at Creation. I hope you understand, as I have learned, the real solution to the health-care dilemma was given long ago.

Chapter 10

Day 4—You've Got Rhythm

And God said, "Let there be lights in the expanse of the sky to separate the day from the night, and let them serve as signs to mark seasons and days and years, and let them be lights in the expanse of the sky to give light on the earth." And it was so. . . . And there was evening, and there was morning—the fourth day (Genesis 1:14-19).

David was prepared and knew about the fourth day of Creation week when we next met. "How in the world does the fourth day relate to my health?" he asked. I was inwardly pleased he was taking a genuine interest. "Doctor Marcum, I just can't see how the sun and stars are a part of God's Health Plan." He was reading his Bible. A relationship was forming. God was getting through to him. I must admit this was exciting to me.

Earth is a solar-powered world, enjoying 98 percent of its warmth from that bright, round orb rising in the east and setting in the west. That endless solar power lifts clouds, pushes the wind, and generates photosynthesis in the plants that feed all living things.

Sunlight also kills germs, boosts your spirit, and enhances your health in ways that are only now becoming known. It is a source of tremendous energy.

So, what do we do? We hide from it! We cover ourselves, shielding our skin from the sun's rays, lathering on chemicals designed to assure us no UV particle worth its salt will get past our oily defenses. We wear hats, sunglasses, and long-sleeved shirts. We pull the curtains, close the shades, and illuminate our homes and offices with artificial sources. The sun has become a boiling bogeyman trying to hunt us down and steal our health with its cancer-producing brilliance.

One problem. History does not record a single civilization dying off because they allowed the sun to shine unencumbered on their cities and homes. Not one moldy, handwritten historical document hiding in a library somewhere includes these words: "The people died off because they failed to apply sunscreen." Instead, there is ample record of people not only embracing the sun, but worshipping it!

So, how did we end up where we are today—thinking the sun is something to be feared instead of worshipped?

Dr. Michael Holick, professor of medicine, physiology, and biophysics at Boston University Medical Center, pulls the curtain back on a medical deception I think is downright criminal. In his book *The UV Advantage* he writes: "The simple answer lies in the fact that there are many billions of dollars to be made in emphasizing the only major medical downside of sun exposure (nonmelanoma skin cancer) and not much money to be made in promoting the sun's many benefits. . . . The major culprits are the cosmetic wing of the pharmaceutical industry and some dermatologists."

Wow! He goes on to say the anti-sun lobby is so desperate to convince you of the sun's dangers and your need to buy their products, "its representatives will tell you with a straight face if it is February in Boston and you are planning to walk to the corner store to buy a quart of milk or sit outside on your lunch break, you should wear sunscreen."

Jerry

Jerry lives as many of us live, in an *indoor* world. He sleeps in a house, drives to town in a tightly sealed automobile, works in a building, grabs a bite to eat at a nearby restaurant, and spends his free time watching television or hunched over the hobby table in his den. His time outdoors is brief and purposeful. Little did he know his "shaded" life was affecting his health and causing many of the symptoms—chest pains, lack of sound sleep, muscle weakness, hypertension, the beginning stages of osteoporosis—that he presented to me on his first visit.

Jerry, like so many of us, is missing a vital element in God's Health Plan. The sun shining down on us was not put there so we could find our way to Walmart without a flashlight. It is a foundational step in gaining and maintaining optimum health—including the health of your heart. We were made to be outside in the sunlight.

Remember how you felt the last time you spent a day outside with that "dangerous" sun lighting your play or your way? If you simply did what was necessary to keep from getting too much exposure and causing your skin to burn, you felt great, refreshed, invigorated. There is a reason for that.

Receiving adequate sunshine was not a problem for our ancestors. They worked outside, played outside, rode in open carriages or on horseback, and even socialized in outdoor venues such as in parks or beside lakes and rivers. What part of God's plan were they accepting into their lives—a part from which many of us fail to benefit? Two words: vitamin D.

I would like to start a new ad campaign, which announces to the world—in no uncertain terms—sunlight is good. My motto: Got Sun?" I want to tell people sunlight is a biblical prescription that carries a whole lot of science behind it.

Chemical Reactions

Vitamin D, actually a hormone, is needed for many important chemical reactions in the body. A few hours of sunshine each week usually does the trick. Many foods contain, or are fortified with, this important element and there is a wide variety of supplements available for those who live a more "shaded" life. Vitamin D is stored and activated for use in the kidneys, but we must have enough stored for our chemistry to run smoothly.

This hormone helps keep our cells from becoming diseased. In countries with little sunlight—near the North or South poles—there is a higher incidence of type 1 diabetes, rheumatoid arthritis, depression and suicide, multiple sclerosis, osteoporosis, and certain types of cancer. Bottom line: We *must* have enough vitamin D in our body. We each have an elaborate internal mechanism to regulate this hormone, letting me know by simple logic how important it is. Why would the liver, kidneys, and parathyroid glands be involved if the Creator did not have special plans for this particular hormone?

Outdoor Deficiency

In this world of indoor living—especially for the elderly and those who call the far northern or southern latitudes home—vitamin D can be deficient. In this case, supplementation is essential. Most health professionals recommend 2,000 international units (IU) per day.

Scientists also tell us too much calcium and animal protein can lower the amount of activated vitamin D in our systems. We are told that cow's milk is good for you—which it is, if you happen to be a calf. What we do not hear on television is that milk and animal proteins can adversely affect activated vitamin D and its reactions in the body.

Then there is our brain. Serotonin is an important brain messenger or "neurotransmitter." Low serotonin levels have been associated with many conditions, including depression and anxiety. Simply put, low levels of this transmitter put stress on the body. This is a worldwide problem and can include the approximately 19 million Americans who suffer from depression. Nearly the same number of Americans also report experiencing chronic anxiety with low levels of serotonin playing a role.

Here is the connection. Sun exposure generates a natural high by stimulating the release of "feel good" substances in your body such as serotonin, dopamine, and beta-endorphins. All three are dependent on vitamin D to function properly. If we do not get enough sunlight, vitamin D levels are lower, thus decreasing the levels of serotonin. One treatment for depression and anxiety is sunlight. Another is to avoid animal protein.

"So," Jerry said when I finished explaining all of this to him, "what's the bottom line, Doc?"

"Well," I said, "God created the sun for many reasons, one of which is to give us vitamin D. So here is what you need to do. Get outside for at least 15 to 30 minutes three or four days a week. If you ever move to a northern latitude, you might want to supplement with 2,000 IUs of vitamin D each day. And keep in mind, adequate vitamin D protection requires exposure to sunlight for only one fourth of the time that is required to burn the skin.

"Use common sense," I added. "Modest tanning is protective, sort of like putting sunglasses on your skin. Just do not overdo." Then I added with a smile, "And just do not *underdo*, either, OK?"

Jerry left my office, not with a prescription needed to be filled at the local drugstore, but with one that can be satisfied with a walk around the neighborhood on a sunny day or an inexpensive supplement. Sorry, drug companies.

As I write this chapter, I cannot help thinking, *How many other chemical reactions are going awry of which we are not even aware—or ever will be aware—simply because we are not following the principles established by our Master Designer?* Why should I turn my back on His instructions when, by all accounts, they have to be irrefutably correct? In the very first chapter of the very first book of His Holy Word, I find His Health Plan in a complete and ready-to-use form. God knows how many hairs are on my head. Wouldn't He also know how to take care of not only my hairy head, but also every other part of my body?

The world and its profit-seeking institutions want the subject of health to be difficult so you and I will pay them big bucks to try to make us well. God's prescriptions for most chronic illnesses are free to everyone and are available everywhere. In my opinion, that is the best deal under the sun.

Moonlighting

There was another "light in the expanse of the sky" making its appearance on day 4 of Creation week. The moon, hanging silently over the land, became the official guardian of night, softly reflecting the sun's rays down onto the newly created plains and lofty mountains.

As far as I can tell, there is no medicinal power generated by moonlight unless you call romance medicinal. But what the moon represents should be of extreme interest to us. God created the day-night cycle on that fourth day—a light-dark system that repeats itself every 24 hours. Suddenly, our world had rhythm, as if some unseen clock had begun to tick in the universe, marking hours of daylight followed by hours of nighttime. For some reason, the Creator knew you and I would need this rhythm in our lives. Today, we know why. We have even given it a name—*circadian* rhythm.

In our modern world, we always seem to be on the go. There are more and more demands on our time. There is always a meeting to attend, tons of e-mails, piles of paper in our in-box, a busy social schedule to maintain, and a home life filled with responsibilities. I have even seen vacationers checking in with the home office by cell phone as they attempt to jam beach umbrellas, coolers, and kids into the family Volvo. We cram more and more into each 24-hour period, even trying to extend daylight by changing how we mark time twice a year. The moon, hovering patiently overhead, is totally ignored, lost in the blaze of streetlights, indoor illumination, and the steady glow of television and computer screens.

In the early part of the nineteenth century, we Americans enjoyed about nine hours of sleep each night. Today, the average is down to seven hours—or less. And exactly what type of sleep are we getting? Every night we allow ourselves to get overstimulated by watching increasingly violent and often downright gross television programs, eating large meals, consuming caffeine-laced drinks and other stimulants, or staying on the job until exhaustion drives us home.

What happened to God's rhythm? What happened to that day-night cycle that was created for a reason? Just think for a moment, we were designed to work taking care of the earth when the sun was up and go to bed when the sun went down. We are ignoring this, bypassing it—totally rejecting the notion such cycles exist. And we are doing so at our own peril.

As a cardiologist, I know rest is definitely a crucial treatment for cardiovascular disease. In the "old days" we frequently demanded bed rest after a heart attack. We need to rest in order to restore worn-out cells—and when I say rest, I mean *sleep*. We need a break from the constant sensory input that is bombarding us. During true rest—the type that takes place in a darkened room with our eyes closed and the covers tucked comfortably under our chins—our stress hormones, which include epinephrine and cortisol, diminish.

While we sleep, increased activity of special white blood cells called "natural killer" cells enhances our immune system and its ability to fight foreign substances such as viruses, bacteria, and even some cancer cells.

Our cortisol levels drop during the night. Cortisol is associated with many disease conditions.

Adequate sleep also helps build and maintain the neurotransmitters of the brain. Have you ever been sleep deprived and noticed how hard it is to think? Within our brains are special chemicals that enable communication with every cell of the body. When these chemicals are disrupted, this communication network is compromised. Without good communication, the function of cells is suboptimal. Sometimes even depression and anxiety may result. During sleep, a growth hormone is secreted—another important chemical for our well-being.

The point I am trying to make is that adequate sleep assists *all* the functions of the body. When lack of rest alters the balance, a whole cascade of events may follow. If one chemical goes up, another chemical might go down, and the results can be anything but pleasant.

Back in the Rhythm

Don't you think it's time to get back into the rhythm God created on the fourth day? Don't you think it's time to stop fighting a rather obvious natural law that includes the sun and the moon as reminders of its presence in our lives?

Or, we could take pills. The drug industry hopes you will make this choice. They will be happy to sell you stimulants and relaxants to get you through your days and nights. They will be more than happy to set you up with stomach pills that mask the fact the meal you ate late in the evening is still hanging around in the morning when you "wake up" from what they tell you is a "good night's rest" when it was nothing more than a drug-induced stupor void of the benefits of true sleep. They will also not refuse to take your money as you battle the many illnesses that lack of sleep brings to the body. They probably have just the thing to address all those side effects from the stimulants and relaxants they sold you. No, they are not breaking any law by making these drugs available to you. It is you who is the lawbreaker, turning your back on one of God's natural laws of health—sleep. But, now you know better. Now *you're* in charge of your health.

In the treatment of all disease, rest and sleep are crucial. Ask yourself, "Do I get better gas mileage when I drive my car at 50 mph or 80 mph? If I owned a champion racehorse, would I run the animal race after race without allowing it to rest between events? Aren't I more important to my family, friends, and coworkers than a car or a horse?"

Do not be deceived into living a life devoid of good rest and sound sleep. Do not think just because you can, you should. God placed the sun and the moon in the heavens as a reminder that while activity and work are essential to good health, so are rest and sleep. When you see that big round moon hovering overhead, do what you were designed to do. Turn off the TV and the computer, put the phone on the machine, and turn out the lights. Let the moon guard your rest as your body takes advantage of that vital downtime to heal, rebuild, and prepare you for the day ahead.

Sleep tight!

Chapter 11

Day 5—A New Song to Sing

And God said, "Let the water teem with living creatures, and let birds fly above the earth across the expanse of the sky." So God created the great creatures of the sea and every living and moving thing with which the water teems, according to their kinds. . . . And God saw that it was good. God blessed them and said, "Be fruitful and increase in number and fill the water in the seas, and let the birds increase on the earth." And there was evening, and there was morning—the fifth day (Genesis 1:20-23).

There are several things I find interesting in the biblical account of day 5 of Creation week—and they all pertain to our health.

First, I am so thankful God created birds and aquatic creatures on that day.

Can you imagine a walk in a forest devoid of birds? Think about it. You hear the wind in the trees and the soft crunch of your shoes on the leafy floor. But that's all. No laughing crows, no chirping chickadees, no trilling wood thrushes, no hooting owls. It would be like listening to a symphony played only by kettledrums with the occasional wood block thrown in.

The second surprising element of the account is found in these words: "God blessed them and said, 'Be fruitful and increase in number.'" OK. God was talking to fish. How do we know this? There was no one else to hear, except the birds. Adam and Eve would not show up until the next day. Nature hears the voice of God.

So, here we have the Creator God making it clear to the birds of the air and the fish of the sea just what they are supposed to do now that they are here. They are supposed to make more birds and fish.

When you look at the very first words of the above quote, you will notice something else. God "blessed" them.

In biblical language, a blessing is a conferring of purpose. Dads blessed their sons, priests blessed their congregations, and prophets blessed entire nations. In each instance, it was made clear, through the blessing, the recipients were given a special responsibility, goal, or position in society.

I find it hard to believe that, when God held His little seashore conference with the fish of the sea and the birds of the air, He was telling them their main purpose in life was to be food. Death and the consumption of animals came later. In Eden, birds and fish were to be on equal standing with all living creatures. They had purpose. They were blessed.

Making Music

Since I do not live underwater, I cannot speak to the full benefit aquatic creatures can bring to our lives, although they sure do a terrific job of keeping our oceans in good repair. A body of water devoid of fish is called "dead" for a reason. Not much of anything else grows there.

But, I can talk about how birds impact a person's health—especially his or her heart. It has to do with music.

Much of what we know regarding how to make melodies and harmonies we learned from the birds. They taught us phrasing, intonation, and breath control. More than one great master of music has left a forest with a tune echoing in his or her head that will become a soul-stirring symphony. And when we hear played or sung notes moving among the scales and hear other notes supporting them, something happens in us—something amazing.

It has been long known music can have a healing effect. This is the biblical treatment for depression and loneliness suggested by David in the Psalms when he spoke of singing a new song (Psalm 149). He took his cue from the birds, and then added trumpets, lutes, harps, stringed instruments, and his own voice (Psalm 150). Whenever David was down, he knew a song of praise would lift him right back up.

All living creatures brought into existence during Creation week were designed to sing praises. Even whales sing. Why? Because God inhabits the praises of His creatures. The bird sitting outside your window on a spring morning is delivering a tune God placed in its mind. The whale drifting among the shadows of the deep is calling out to its mate in a voice created by God Himself. When the angels announced Christ's birth, they did not go around mumbling under their breaths or writing out paper invitations. They sang. They sang loud and clear! Their music filled the countryside and moved the hearts of simple shepherds.

Music can calm the stresses of life. When a baby needs to go to sleep, we sing a lullaby. When we are worried or concerned, many of us hum softly to ourselves. The next time you watch a television program with a scene centered on true love and gentle compassion, listen to the supporting music. It is soft, rich, and soothing. Music is a powerful force for healing.

Medical Treatment

I was listening to the Wedgewood Trio and praying for the right words to place in this chapter about music as a medical treatment. The Wedgewood Trio is made up of three musicians who have been playing and singing together since the 1960s. One plays an upright bass, the second a guitar, and the third alternates through several instruments, including a harmonica.

They have always performed songs filled with praise and hope. As I listened to their beautiful melodies and harmonies, I found myself beginning to relax. My heart rate and breathing slowed. A peace came over me. I believe the Holy Spirit filled my mind with thoughts and scenes I needed to include in this chapter. I found, just like the birds of Eden, that music offered a special way of preparing me to commune with the One who made me, a special aspect of worship.

I am not naive enough to think the music I enjoy is the only music God uses to touch hearts. Making or hearing music is very individualized. Sometimes, to bring about His purpose, there may be no instrument or voice involved at all. Some find healing in the whisper of the wind as it moves through the trees. For others, it might be the ocean's roar that brings peace to their soul. It could be chirping birds or buzzing insects that lower the blood pressure and slow the heart of still others. That is why all nature sings some type of song. They sing for a reason. They, as we, were designed to praise God through their song. If you are like me, your favorite type of music might include the absolute stillness at the end of a hectic day.

What matters is the heart of the musician. What matters is the source of the song.

Like everything else God created, deceptions have mutated the music of this world. The wrong type of music can damage our chemistry, causing our bodies to respond in unhealthy ways. Some very heinous crimes have been committed while loud, dissonant music was blaring from nearby boom boxes or on the family stereo. There is a reason that many soldiers go into battle with loud, strident tunes playing in their earbuds.

Dissonant tunes, boom boxes, and heinous crimes did not exist in Eden when God called the birds into being. The song He gave them to sing—the song with which He blessed them—was simple and beautiful. It was a melody continually filling their hearts with joy and praise.

We were made to praise God in song, and when we do, we are following the Owner's Manual even if we do not understand the exact physiology as of this writing. Music can be more powerful than a pill.

When was the last time you felt poorly after singing a song of praise to God? That is not going to happen. There is a chemical reaction behind that good feeling. When David needed a lift, he sang. When the birds wanted to respond to God's love on that fifth day of Creation, they sang.

The music is in you. The blessing has already been given. The healing is waiting to happen. Sing!

Chapter 12

Day 6—Someone to Love

And God said, "Let the land produce living creatures according to their kinds: livestock, creatures that move along the ground, and wild animals, each according to its kind." And it was so. . . . Then God said, "Let us make man in our image, in our likeness, and let them rule over the fish of the sea and the birds of the air, over the livestock, over all the earth, and over all the creatures that move along the ground." So Go created man in his own image. . . . And there was evening, and there was morning—the sixth day (Genesis 1:24-31).

As I entered the room, my hand was barely off the doorknob when David exclaimed, "Doctor Marcum, I know exactly why day 6 is in God's Health Plan. I figured it out all by myself just by reading the Bible and praying. I didn't need *Wikipedia*, a library, or theologian. You are right. The Bible can be 'figured out' by a guy like me." Inwardly, I knew David would need me less and less now. God was talking directly to his heart.

The sixth day of Creation was a busy one by any standard. Imagine the work that would go into creating—from scratch mind you—an elephant. Where do you put everything? Or how about a cat? Or a zebra? Think of the creative power necessary to form a single, living ant. Amazing!

Then there's man. This creature would enjoy the added benefit of being able to be innovative and generate technology to help people live better lives, build skyscrapers, airplanes, and cell phones. Man would be able to think and reason in ways the animals could not. And—this is important to remember— man was created in the image of God Himself. He was unique, special, and highly intelligent, and for all intents and purposes, godlike.

After Adam was created, God made it very clear what He had in mind as far as man's relationship with animals is concerned. "Now the Lord God

. . . brought [the animals] to the man to see what he would name them; and whatever the man called each living creature, that was its name. So the man gave names to all the livestock, the birds of the air and all the beasts of the field" (Genesis 2:19).

Let me ask you a question. What happens when you name a stray dog or cat that appears at your doorstep? That's right, it becomes something special to you. In your mind, it belongs to you. It is part of your world. In short, you begin to love it.

That is exactly what God could have had in mind when He asked Adam to name every living creature on this earth. He wanted him to experience that sense of ownership, of responsibility, of love so that when he ruled over the animal kingdom, every decision he made concerning God's creatures would flow from a heart filled with respect and a deep commitment to each animal's safety and comfort. Not exactly the image coming to mind when you think of the way we treat animals today. They are being used as a food source for much of the world. Even domesticated creatures are rounded up and put in "animal shelters," and if no one claims them, well, you get the picture. God's Health Plan took into consideration the well-being of both humans *and animals.*

Healing Pets

The health benefits of people interacting—in a loving, supportive way—with animals are well documented. One study suggests spending a little time with the family pet may relieve greater amounts of stress than taking a pill, talking with a best friend, or even conversing with your spouse.

Sometimes, it seems, animals can even work miracles. Consider this from a recent ABC News report. A golden retriever called Janie walked down the hall of the Cedars-Sinai Medical Center in Los Angeles and breezed into the room of a patient who had refused to talk to anyone in weeks. Then Janie did something the best medical treatments had been unable to do. As she put her paws on the edge of the bed, the patient leaned over, began stroking her ears, and started talking.

Researchers across the country are discovering that pets can do everything from reducing blood pressure during times of intense stress to easing the pain of loneliness.

Animals are even therapeutic for people with Alzheimer's, says Dr. John W. Tracy, a family practice physician in Fancy Gap, Virginia, because they get people to look inside themselves a little bit.

A study was done at Purdue University in which researchers examined the effect of a fish tank on patients with Alzheimer's. Before the fish tank, many patients at a particular nursing home were wandering away from the table during meals, reducing the amount of nutrition they received. But after the staff installed an aquarium in the dining room and stocked it with colorful fish, patients remained in their seats and ate their entire meals in peace.

Sarah

Sarah had been my patient for four years. I was treating her for atrial fibrillation—a condition in which the upper chamber of the heart beats rapidly. She had done well with the treatment, and we both were encouraged.

During this time I had also gotten to know her husband, Mac. Mac loved two things: driving his truck and caring for Sarah. They always came to the office together and were obviously very much in love.

One day Mac became sick with pneumonia and died suddenly at the age of 82. When Sarah came back to visit a month after the funeral, she seemed totally and understandably lost. She was a woman of faith and turned to God for help, but still carried a broken heart. Her blood pressure was up, she was not sleeping well at night, and her memory was beginning to slip. Her family was supporting her, but without the love of her life, her health was fading.

I had seen this before. When a loved one passes, the stress from the loss places an extreme burden on a body. If something is not done quickly, damage can result. Yes, people can die of a broken heart.

One of my patients had an extra dog and I suggested to Sarah she adopt this lovable ball of fur. Three months passed, and when my patient came in for her quarterly checkup, she was a completely different woman. Sarah told me about her new Maltese, and though she still missed Mac, she had learned to love that dog, and the pooch had responded with an overflow of love in return. I was not surprised. Animals—as designed by God—can help our chemistry by giving us unconditional love.

I experience this with my own dogs, Max and Daphne. My wife really does not care for them when they insist on doing their business in the house, but whenever I come home from work, they are always there to greet me—making me feel like I am the most important human in the world. When I must stay up late at night, they patiently sit at my feet. Max and Daphne lower my stress levels by showing me love.

Animals enrich our lives—amaze us, cheer us up, calm us down, allay our fears, and bring our world to life. That was the Creator's intent when He made them for us to enjoy. A large part of God's Health Plan includes friendly, loving interaction with *all* the creatures of this world. In fact, we are all healers when we make someone laugh, feel good about themselves, or show them love. We change their chemistry for the good. Animals are prescriptions for the world, and we too can be a prescription for the world.

But, God had one more healthy surprise waiting for Adam on that sixth day of Creation. That's right. Eve!

Here is an interesting fact. Married people tend to live longer and healthier than single people. Perhaps I had better restate that with one word added. *Happily* married people tend to live longer and healthier than their single friends. Scientists conclude it probably has to do with the lowering of stress that comes when a person's heart is filled with love; when the focus is on someone other than yourself; when you have someone with whom to share life's ups and downs. Whatever the reason, God created the institution of marriage for our health. It is part of His plan.

And, where there is marriage, more than likely, there is family.

Matthew

Matthew had been in the intensive care for a week when I got to know him. He was 54 and suffered from an infection on his leg—a condition that began on a camping trip the month before. He didn't pay much attention to it at first.

This infection did not clear up. One of the predisposing conditions that made him more susceptible was the fact Matthew was a diabetic. Diabetes inhibits the immune system. The infection moved from the leg into the bloodstream, and he became very sick with high temperatures and low blood pressure. The infection also damaged the mitral valve in his heart and caused a dangerous leak. Because fluid was building up in his lungs, he was put on the ventilator and, as quickly as possible, surgery was scheduled to replace the leaky valve. We all feared that he would die. The numbers did not look good. Even though we had done everything we could, we honestly did not know if he would pull through.

One thing I did notice about Matthew was that he had a very strong family. The kids, his wife, the in-laws, his mom and dad, they were all there supporting him, praying for him, helping in any way possible, showing their love and concern.

I believe there is healing power in family because the original social unit on this earth—the original human structure God set up in Eden—was the family. Adam had Eve. Eve had Adam. In time, there would be little Adams and Eves running around, filling their lives with happy laughter. Love would spread from person to person. But that was just the beginning.

The family was also designed to be the place to worship and learn about God, to help each other survive and make a living, to belong, and, after deception entered the world, provide a safe harbor in which to weather the stresses of life.

Matthew enjoyed this type of environment, and I believe this aided his healing. No, I cannot measure its effect on paper or chart the results on a graph, but it was real, and my patient's ability to survive such a stressful ordeal is proof in so many cases, family makes a healing difference.

Unfortunately, there is a deception in the world that says, "Family is not all that important. Kids do not need a mom *and* a dad. Hey, you can have it all—a career, a big home, and a loving family." In the midst of this lie, the divorce rate is rising. Families are dissolving right before our eyes, and society is suffering untold misery because of it.

In this fast-paced world, we are forgetting the healing power of family. This is where love is learned, where God is revealed, where worship is expressed. When He came to this earth, Christ spent more time in a family unit than He did in active ministry. During this family time, He was learning and growing. When His work finally did begin, He had the tools and support network necessary to keep Him going in the face of agonizing barriers. How many young people can say the same thing about their family structure today?

I will bet you never thought of family as a treatment for disease. Well, it is. A good family will change our chemistry. When this precious, healing unit is torn apart, we have a much harder time learning about love the way God intended.

One More Thing

So, here we are, six days into Creation week. Adam and Eve are standing, hand in hand, surveying all that God has done, and reveling in the beauty and majesty of every tree, flower, and animal. They are breathing deeply of the nature-scented air, drinking from pure, sparkling streams, eating of the fresh fruits and vegetables growing in abundance all around them. What more could they possibly need?

That is when God spoke again. We do not know what words He used, but His meaning was clear. "The Lord God took the man and put him in the Garden of Eden to work it and take care of it" (Genesis 2:15).

Work? Did God just instruct Adam and Eve to work? Why? They had everything they needed: a beautiful garden home, food, fellowship with each other and the animals! Why work?

Because God knew physical activity—especially physical activity resulting in a feeling of accomplishment or satisfaction—is good for your health. Activity is also good for your brain. Mentally active people tend to enjoy an increased clarity of thought well into old age. Spiritually active folk, who attend church regularly, volunteer, get involved with the needs of others, tend to remain closer to God as the years roll by.

Yes, God created us with legs instead of roots for a reason. We were designed to move and be active while taking care of the earth. Over the course of centuries, especially the past 50 years, we have been moving less and less. Such inactivity is taking a tremendous chemical toll on our bodies.

Chemical toll? That is right. Activity enables our body to make chemicals, which help lower our blood pressure, strengthen our immune system, and make our bones stronger. It helps us burn fat—a growing concern in this country where obesity rates are skyrocketing. As a matter of fact, fat has its own scientific name now. It is called the endocannabinoid system. This system is capable of making chemicals of its own—chemicals that damage the body. The fat we are carrying around seems to have a life of its own! Activity, exercise, movement—whatever you want to call it—helps prevent the endocannabinoid system from stressing the body.

Sam

Sam ventured into my office a few years ago. He weighed in at 400 pounds and stood five and a half feet tall. I knew right away his endocannabinoid system, i.e., body fat, was changing him chemically. His blood sugar was high. He had elevated blood pressure and suffered from diabetes.

The burden of carrying around the extra weight was causing his joints to painfully give out. Because of all his prescriptions, he was suffering from numerous side effects—impotence being one of them. In short, Sam felt lousy.

He is not alone. Up to 60 percent of Americans are overweight, and the industrialized world is also "growing" at similar rates.

I explained to Sam that too many calories and too little exercise over a period of time was his true enemy. Excess fat causes the body to work harder. This raises blood pressure, increases the workload on the heart, elevates cholesterol levels, and multiplies the chance of developing diabetes. Fat causes the body to handle sugar incorrectly, creating extra insulin, which is not a good thing either.

"What do you mean?" he asked.

"Well," I continued, "insulin is a substance that helps sugar move into the body's cells. High levels of blood sugar may also cause the blood pressure to increase. The increased amount of fat causes the liver to handle fats abnormally, turning fat into artery-clogging cholesterol. And not only does the risk of cardiovascular disease increase; the risk of cancer and asthma skyrockets as well. Women who gain more than 20 pounds after the age of 18 double the risk of postmenopausal breast cancer. Every two pounds of extra weight increases the risk of arthritis by at least 9 percent. Bottom line, Sam? All of the diseases with which you are suffering from are really symptoms of being overweight. If you lose the weight, you will lose the symptoms."

Sam's mouth dropped open. "No one has ever put it to me like that," he said. "Do you think a weight loss pill would help?"

I explained to Sam we are being deceived by all the many diets and weight loss plans out there. These can be expensive and dangerous. "There are no quick fixes," I told him. "As a matter of fact, some diet pills have caused major health issues. Many of the diets and exercise plans just leave a person unhappy and stressed out. A person spends a lot of money, loses a bit of weight, then quickly gains it back again. And another cycle begins."

I could not help feeling the pain and frustration my patient was feeling. Sam, like many of us, wanted a quick fix. He wanted more medication to help with his symptoms. But I knew he would be back in my office within months—possibly with even more health problems. "If you really want to feel better," I told him, "you're going to have to start living better. It's a journey, not a destination. Are you serious about this, because I sure am?"

Sam nodded. "Just tell me what I have to do, Doctor Marcum."

Together, we worked out a plan—a health plan for Sam.

He could barely walk across the room when we started. So we set small but important goals. At first he walked one minute a couple times a day. That's right. One minute. Then we began to increase his walk time to five minutes, then 10, then 20. In a matter of weeks, he began to feel better and we took him off a blood pressure medication.

Next, Sam's walk spanned 30 minutes, then 40 minutes a day. He started to feel even better and the dose of his diabetes medications was lowered.

He began to walk faster and added some light strength training. His chemistry responded in some amazing ways as he experienced undeniable proof we were designed to be active.

Other changes occurred as well. Now, after four years, Sam does 45 minutes of aerobic exercises with 20 minutes of strength training six days a week. Then he takes one day a week off to rest. He has lost 200 pounds, no longer has high blood pressure, is not diabetic, suffers fewer joint pains, is not depressed, and does not stagger under the debilitating side effects of medications. Actually, he now takes one medication—for his seasonal allergies.

Today, how many doctors include on their prescription tablets the word "walk"? How many sit down with their patients and outline a workable walking program? Some do. But most, I am afraid, would say, "Who has time for that?"

God knew exactly what we needed. The antidote for so many of the diseases from which we suffer today was staring Adam and Eve squarely in the face. "Here is your garden," the Creator told them. "Tend it. Care for it. Keep moving. Keep working. Be active!"

We may not be tending gardens these days, but the principle remains. We were not meant to sit and stare and be inactive. We were made to move. It is part of the plan.

The Bridge

I recall a story told to me by a crew member who worked for Faith for Today, a Christian television ministry. The production team was in San Francisco filming a documentary on the subject of suicide. Now, don't get me wrong. The hardworking folk who live in San Francisco are not suicide-prone. That is not why the crew was there. It's *what's* in San Francisco that drew the filmmakers to that part of California.

Stretching majestically over the inlet leading to that beautiful bay is the Golden Gate Bridge, a marvel of engineering and, apparently, a powerful magnet for people who want to end their lives.

While the crew was setting up their equipment in order to interview one of the security guards at the entrance to the bridge, the scanner in the guard booth rattled to life. "Attention all security personnel. We've got a jumper mid-span. I repeat. We've got a jumper mid-span." Sure enough, while the Faith for Today production team was getting ready to talk with a guard about the many suicides on the bridge, a small, foreign-built car stopped in the middle of the center span. The driver, a young man wearing worn jeans and a T-shirt, had unhurriedly exited the vehicle, walked to the railing, climbed to the upper pole, hesitated for just a moment, then stepped out into space. His life ended with a silent splash far below.

In his car he had left a note with these words carefully written across its wrinkled surface: "Happiness is someone to love, something to do, and something to look forward to."

On the sixth day of Creation, God fulfilled all three of these requirements for Adam and Eve. He gave them someone to love. He showed them a garden waiting to be tended and a world filled with animals eager for attention and care so they would always have something to do. And, finally, He told them, "Be fruitful and increase in number; fill the earth and subdue it" (Genesis 1:28). Earth's first couple could look forward to becoming earth's first parents—sharing the same flawless creative power that had formed them in the first place.

Biblical scholars will tell you that on the sixth day of Creation week, God made animals and man. This is true. But He set in place the most powerful healing agent this world would ever see. On day 6, God created love.

Chapter 13

Day 7—Healing Rest

By the seventh day God had finished the work he had been doing; so on the seventh day he rested from all his work. And God blessed the seventh day and made it holy, because on it he rested from all the work of creating that he had done (Genesis 2:2, 3).

At the end of a long day's work, American cowboys liked nothing better than to sit by a crackling fire and kick off their boots, eager to savor the coming night's rest. On the seventh day of each week, God invites us to do the same. It is part of His amazing Health Plan.

The word "rested" found in Genesis, chapter 2, verse 1 also means "to cease" or "to stop doing what you have been doing." So, in essence, God stopped working; stopped creating on the seventh day. Today, Christians know that day as the "Sabbath," or "day of rest."

Generations later, from the summit of Mount Sinai, God reminded the children of Israel how He wanted the holy day observed. Listen to His words as recorded in Exodus 20, starting with verse 8. "Remember the Sabbath day by keeping it holy. Six days you shall labor and do all your work, but the seventh day is a Sabbath to the Lord your God. On it you shall not do any work. . . . For in six days the Lord made the heavens and the earth, the sea, and all that is in them, but he rested on the seventh day. Therefore the Lord blessed the Sabbath day and made it holy."

I do not know how you feel about this, but it seems to me God is demonstrating a genuine concern about how we spend our Sabbath hours. By using the word "remember," He indicated that this was a part of the original health plan, which could easily be forgotten. Resting is often not equated with a change in the body's chemistry or even a treatment for ailments. Resting is required for the maintenance of the entire system. As I tell my patients, you get better gas mileage when you drive at 50 rather than 80 miles an hour. At the end of Creation week God was concerned for our future health.

Today, scientists are discovering an interesting fact. Rest—or ceasing from our labors—is not only good for our minds; it is incredibly good for our bodies as well.

In our fast-paced, exhausting lives, insomnia is running rampant. People are gulping down millions of sedatives and tranquilizers, desperate for the rest that can restore their energies. Those who take no relief from the daily grind suffer increased bouts of cold and flu and are often depressed. They become irritable, lose their tempers more often, and even the simplest tasks seem overwhelming. Without providing your mind and body sufficient rest, burnout waits just around the corner. Being sleep or rest deprived turns on the stress cascade we have mentioned, not good over the long haul.

You see, when God was creating this world, He was looking beyond the needs of Adam and Eve. Using His incredible mind of love, He was scanning the future, visualizing you and me languishing in a world overtaken by deceptions. He saw our need to escape from the pain of life; from the hurt and sorrow He knew we might be facing. So, on the last day of Creation week, He became an example for us to learn from—a perfect template around which we could fashion our lives. On the seventh day, God rested. And so should we.

Rest means a lot more than *sleep*. It is a day made holy by the Creator in which we should change our focus, slow our pace, and redirect our motivations. It is a day in which we can stop worrying about ourselves and spend time serving others. How? Many find opportunities for rest by attending church, listening to God speak to them in sermons, getting involved in outreach programs, singing in the choir, teaching our children, or greeting visitors at the door.

Others seek the solitude of nature: roaming forest paths or walking deserted beaches. Some spend the hours of the Sabbath reading, or listening to inspiring music. There are many ways to rest on God's holy day. And, yes, if that is what is needed, some close their eyes and sleep, spending hours cradled by the knowledge they are giving their bodies the much-needed opportunity to recharge.

Rest, in all forms, allows the body to renew itself. It aids in the healing of injuries and infections—including emotional traumas. Rest strengthens the body's immune system, helping to protect against disease. And proper rest can actually add length to life. Is it any wonder that God created a day of rest; that He included rest in His original Health Plan?

Some people say I have an active imagination, and perhaps I do. But there is an image I like to form in my mind when I see the sun slipping below the horizon at the end of the sixth day of the week. I form a picture of Jesus standing above the setting sun, arms outstretched, looking right at me. From His lips I hear His words recorded in Matthew 11, starting with verse 28. "Come to me, all you who are weary and burdened, and I will give you rest. Take my yoke upon you and learn from me, for I am gentle and humble in heart, and you will find rest for your souls."

I invite you to try resting one day a week. While God loves to be worshipped on any day of the week and eagerly looks forward to spending time with you, He specifically asked us to work six days and rest a day. He could have worked two and rested one or worked nine and rested one, but the Creator knew this was how He designed us to function optimally, work six days and rest. There is only one day He set aside as holy; only one day He included in His powerful Health Plan. That is the *seventh*-day Sabbath—the one He created way back in Eden designed specifically to nurture and protect our health and well-being.

As a behavioral cardiologist, I can say from experience rest is definitely a treatment for cardiovascular disease. We need rest to restore our bodies and replace worn-out and dead cells. We need a break from all the sensory input that constantly bombards us. During physical rest, our stress hormones diminish.

Not only do I believe in physical rest, but I also believe in a mental rest, during which we renew the spiritual component of our lives. Would God be giving us a principle not beneficial for our long-term health?

Kaye

Kaye appeared in my office as winter was fading into the expectations of spring. At 52, her olive skin showed few wrinkles. Her intelligent green eyes shone with a hint of hope as she began telling me the reason for her visit to the mountains of eastern Tennessee, far from her home on the Eastern Shore of Maryland. At five feet eight inches in height, she boasted an athletic build. One would never know she had been ill for many years.

Kaye carried a strong family history of heart disease. She experienced her first bypass surgery at 43 and a repeat performance at 50. As I looked through her well-organized records, I noticed she had already seen some of the most respected cardiologists in the country. She was already receiving every possible, scientifically proven treatment and was coming to me, as many patients do, for a second opinion; to see if anything else could be offered to improve her condition.

As we visited, I discovered a little bit more about her. She had smoked cigarettes throughout her 20s but had kicked that habit completely. Now she operated a very successful business keeping her traveling much of the time. Her two children attended college and her husband, an attorney, maintained an equally demanding career. She admitted she rarely did anything "just for Kaye."

My visitor was on all the right medications at the correct dosages. Her blood pressure, cholesterol levels, and diet were exemplary, and she exercised 45 minutes a day. But she still felt miserable much of the time.

Finally, to make sure all the bases were covered, I began to explore how much time she spent in rest. I knew lack of rest is a gigantic stressor that is often overlooked. She seemed puzzled and a little surprised as I probed this aspect of her life. Sensing her unspoken questions, I began to explain why I wanted to know about her rest patterns.

The Hidden Culprit

When God created the universe, He also designed certain laws that would govern its operation. Sir Isaac Newton was the first to clearly explain one such principle. It dictates if you jump off a cliff, there will be severe consequences. This law remains in full force whether you believe in it or not. Gravity is well known to any child who has ever tried to fly.

I explained to Kaye, just as there are laws that hold the universe together, there are certain laws governing how well our bodies function. One of those irrefutable, seldom recognized, yet extremely powerful laws is rest. Like gravity, you ignore it at your own peril.

I told my visitor our bodies, when healthy, maintain a certain chemical profile—just enough of this, just enough of that. But the profile is not static. It changes to meet demands. If you get an infection, the body heats itself up to kill the germs. When you sit in the sun too long, the body releases moisture to cool off. When the mind senses danger, the body prepares to either face the foe or get out of Dodge . . . fast. Most of what happens in the body takes place as the result of changes in its chemistry, which, in many cases, is a good thing.

However, infections and creeping tigers are not the only foes we face. Work-, environment-, or relationship-related stresses, chronic illnesses, malnutrition brought on by unhealthy food choices, lack of adequate water intake, a sedentary lifestyle, even watching the six-o'clock news can alter our chemistry in some rather profound ways. Our body, sensing the strain, tries to meet the demand by making adjustments. In the case of illness, the body does what it needs to do to bring about healing, which may include shutting down or altering some important bodily functions. In other words, the body is trying to meet the challenge, and then return to a balanced state as quickly as possible.

But, what if the challenge is never-ending? What if the stress continues day after day, week after week, year after year? The body remains in an altered, unbalanced state, its chemistry profile far from the status quo—like operating a car with its brakes on or trying to build a house without adequate tools or materials.

This brought us back to the law of rest. Rest is an important factor in "resetting" the body; allowing it to return to a more balanced condition. Without an adequate and regular release from the tensions of everyday challenges, our chemistry begins to change for the worse.

As I continued, I could tell that I had sparked Kaye's interest. She was especially intrigued when I posed this rhetorical question: "Would you rather take a prescription medication to change your chemistry, or would you like to learn how to rest and accomplish the same thing and a whole lot more?"

I explained that the God of the universe worked six days when creating this earth. Then He rested the seventh day. He set up this pattern at the beginning. God Himself chose to rest on the seventh day. Did He really need to rest? He even went so far as to bless this rest (Genesis 2:2, 3), setting it aside for a special purpose. Apparently, our Creator understood a ratio of one in seven—one day of rest for six days of honest labor—brought about just the right balance in the human body. That is why He created the law of rest right along with fresh air, pure water, sunlight, palm trees, and aardvarks.

I then reemphasized to Kaye, when we violate one of God's laws—whether we believe the law exists or not—our chemistry is altered. After all, the Creator knows how His creation is supposed to operate. That is why He put His laws into place—the laws of health so many of us ignore, reject, or do not even know about. When we fail to rest, our chemistry—as expected—changes for the worse. As a result, stress is placed on *all* systems of the body.

Cycles of Life

That weekly rest was only part of the picture. As we have mentioned earlier, God also created the day-night cycles we call "circadian rhythms." Every one of us operates under their steady cadence. The body is actually hard-wired to slow down at night and speed up during the day—a cycle determined by one of many hormones, including melatonin and serotonin.

In today's world, this natural rhythm is frequently disrupted. Think of the late-night eating that does not allow our gastrointestinal system to rest. Stimuli such as television, the Internet, iPods, and cell phones constantly bombard our systems long after the sun goes down. Then, because of lack of adequate sleep at night, we chemically stimulate our bodies to keep going the next day. Day after day, week after week, month after month, and year after year, the pattern continues. Sometimes we doze during the day—sometimes with tragic results. When this day-night cycle is compromised, our chemistry is disrupted.

I asked Kaye, "Have you ever been sleep deprived or worked a long time without rest?"

She nodded.

"Well," I continued, "under those conditions, the law of rest is being violated. The physical, emotional, and cognitive functions of the body are compromised. Stress is placed on the entire system."

During these times, our stress chemicals—including epinephrine and cortisol—rise. They, in turn, alter other chemical reactions in the body. If this condition goes on long enough, the body can be eventually damaged by a heart attack, ulcers, poor digestion, tight muscles, high blood pressure, palpitations, headaches, strokes, a weak immune system, and a host of other pains—all because God's law of rest was ignored. Most chronic diseases that plague modern society have stress as a component, which includes the lack of needed rest as a major component.

True Confession

At this point, I asked Kaye rather bluntly, "Have you been violating God's natural law of rest? Are you jumping off a ten-story building?"

I watched my patient closely as a new understanding crept into her mind. It was painfully obvious that I had hit upon an area of her life that she had allowed to become out of control. Gently, I suggested that by making some small but consistent changes in her life, her stress chemistry could greatly improve. If additional and regular rest could be added to her treatment regimen, it just might penetrate to the very core of her problem. "After all," I said, "why would the God of the universe mention rest if it were not important?

"Kaye," I continued, "don't you want the best for your children?"

"Of course," she responded emphatically, unsure of why I had asked such a question.

"Well," I said, learning forward slightly, "God wants the best for you, too."

After a short pause, she looked inquisitively at me with genuine interest. "Doctor Marcum," she said, "I don't mean to put you on the spot, but I really want to know, how does a cardiologist rest?"

With a smile, I explained I try to get adequate sleep at night, though call nights are challenging. I try to faithfully keep to the seven-day cycle God designed. On the seventh day of each week, I try to get more rest—physical and mental. I sleep longer and do my best to not think about my work. I spend time worshipping and listening to the God who created me. I plan special activities for my family, which might include heading to the great outdoors, a special meal, spending time with friends, helping someone in need, or giving an extra measure of love where needed—anything to break my everyday routine.

How people rest, I explained, is personal and depends on their definition of the word. For some, resting is climbing a mountain. For others, it might be snoozing in the shade of a backyard tree. Still others find rest in association with their church family or simply strolling along a deserted beach. The key is to learn how *God* wants you to rest and then stick to it, realizing it is vital to optimal health. Rest is necessary to prevent *and treat* disease.

Our session was coming to an end and I once more explained when we live in harmony with God's laws, our chemistry improves, stress is relieved, and healing can occur. What she needed most was true rest—healing rest—a powerful and gracious gift and prescription from God.

On that late spring day, I believe a new treatment was added to Kaye's regimen, one without adverse side effects and filled with eternal benefits. She left my office with a fresh understanding and a desire to learn more about God's timeless laws for building and maintaining optimum health. Her healing had already begun.

Worship

My conversation with Kaye got me to thinking, not only about rest, but worship as well. Christians tend to spend at least a portion of the holy day, the rest day, engaged in some sort of worship. For many, the homage we pay is not to our Creator, but to something very different—and that difference can take a toll on our health. Let me explain.

Kelli, my 13- going on 20-year-old daughter, asked me why so many people make such a big deal about football and other sports. I must admit, we as a society, myself included, spend considerable time with sports of all sorts. I explained the game is exciting, fun to play and watch, and the competition between equally matched teams allows each player's skills to be put to the test. That is about all I could say. While those of us who love the game see a combination of strategy and strength on the field, all Kelli sees are really big men running into each other and knocking each other down. To a 13-year-old girl, that must seem very strange indeed.

Football also teaches me something about God, and about worship. We have been learning in the last few chapters about biblical treatments to help change our chemistry. Our Creator God is constant. He does not change. The laws He set in motion during Creation week are also constant. Like the coach of a winning football team, it makes perfect sense God would give us the best game plan to care for our bodies. It also makes perfect sense to me that the evil one would target his deceptions at that plan as well.

Which brings me back to worship. While I certainly enjoy a good football game as much as the next guy, I know you and I were not designed to *worship* football—or any other sport for that matter. It seems a little strange to me that, in the fall, hundreds of thousands of people will flock to games each Saturday and Sunday. Not only that, we spend hours watching sports on TV, reading about our favorite teams and players in the newspaper, and listening to guys on the radio go on and on about the next game. Even water-cooler conversations usually focus on sports. Baseball, basketball, Nascar, golf, soccer—the list seems endless. Again, while there is absolutely nothing wrong with these sports per se, there is a problem when they become objects of worship. We were designed to worship our Creator, not some sports team or athlete.

Wouldn't it be great if our places of worship experienced growing attendance, with hundreds of thousands of people paying money, standing in line for hours to pay homage to our Creator? Wouldn't it be great if people wore clothes proclaiming the greatness of God rather than the logo of a local team? What if the seemingly endless talk shows on the radio and television were praising God and talking about how we could enhance our worship of Him? In addition to a sports page in our local newspaper, what if there was a worship page? What if, at the water cooler, we spoke of God and His greatness in our lives, sharing with our coworkers ways to know Him better?

I can answer those "what if" questions. We would be healthier. We would live longer. We would have a lot less stress and diseases in our lives. Why? Because we become like who and what we worship. Our chemistry improves when we shift our focus to the One who designed us. Worship can be a powerful treatment if what we worship fills our hearts with joy and love.

Of course, the evil one wants to discredit the Creation health plan and those who proclaim the chemical importance of worshipping the true God. But we know better. Health has always been, and always will be, about who and what we worship.

"Where Are You?"

I wish I could have been there on the first Sabbath in Eden. If you will allow me one more flight of imagination, I see Adam and Eve strolling through their sunlit garden, marveling at the animals—each of which has been named. They pause and drink deeply from a clear-flowing stream or pluck a brightly colored fruit from an overhanging limb.

They listen to the symphony echoing from the trees as birds fill the air with their praise songs. The grass underfoot is soft and welcoming, and they settle down to nap as the whispering breezes carry them gently into slumber. They feel a deep and safe love for each other and the world they inhabit.

Then they hear a voice calling out to them. "Adam? Eve? Where are you? There are many more beauties I want to show you."

I can hear their expressions of joy as they run into the arms of the Creator Himself. Like children, they follow Him along verdant paths and beside glass-clear lakes, marveling at the amazing sights and sounds at each step, laughing and smiling as God reveals His detailed handiwork.

How is it possible for them to be so happy? Because God's Health Plan is in full force in their lives. They have not allowed anything damaging into their existence—nothing is present that can diminish their vitality. They are healthy in mind, body, and spirit. They are one with the Creator. They are following His Health Plan to the letter.

While it may not be so easy for us today after years of deception, it is still possible to enjoy the incredible benefits God intended for us. His Health Plan still exists, just waiting to bring healing to our bodies and minds.

Chapter 14

The Depth of the Deception

et me get this straight," David said as I closed the Bible and slid it across the desk in his direction. "You're telling me if I don't want to have another heart attack, I've got to become a gardener?"

I couldn't help laughing at his question, even though I sensed a touch of frustration in his voice. "Wouldn't hurt," I responded with a chuckle. "Doesn't pay much, though."

David's eyes narrowed. "That just proves it, Doc," he said. "This Bible—this Owner's Manual as you call it—is nothing but a bunch of fairy tales and outdated concepts that don't make sense in today's world."

"Oh, really?" I asked. "Then how do you explain the fact that many—if not most—of the diseases with which we struggle today became widespread as more and more of us moved from the country into the cities; as we turned our backs on our farms and became apartment dwellers and factory workers? How do you explain that, even today, the healthiest societies are still made up of people who work the land and eat their own harvest—people such as the rural Chinese, Japanese, or Southeast Asians? How do you explain the fact history records the amazing longevity of nations whose people lived off the land—nations such as the ancient Mayans or many African societies? Try to find heart disease in today's African backcountries. Try to find diabetes among the poor farming communities of Asia and South America.

"For that matter," I pressed, "look at North America. Before 1900, our diet consisted mostly of foods grown in local gardens and nearby farms, supplemented with a few choice items from the general store. What meat we did eat on special occasions came from our own barnyard. In 1900, 10 to 15 percent of deaths in the country were from cardiovascular disease. Now, as we move into the twenty-first century—just 100 years later—almost every second death is from heart disease. Even cancer deaths have shot up dramatically in spite of modern medical interventions. David, people did not change. But their lifestyle did, especially when it came to what they dumped down their throats. We have moved from kernels of corn to buckets from the "Colonel." We have traded spring water for soda pop. The whole food nature so willingly provides now has the nutrition processed right out of it and, to make up for the loss of flavor, we pour on sugars, salts, and copious amounts of preservatives to increase shelf life and 'eye-appeal.' I stand by my statement. We could all do a lot worse than becoming gardeners."

David was silent for a long moment. I sensed a crack beginning to form in his outer shell of frustration so I continued, hoping he would allow a few more pieces of the puzzle to fall into place.

Subtle Dangers

I shared with David a small list of dangers to his health of which he—and most of my paitents—are blissfully unaware. These deceptions are literally killing people. I see it every day.

Deception No. 1—Caffeine makes you think better.

Just the opposite is true. Caffeine binds to receptors in the brain, which constrict blood flow. The body, sensing the restriction, responds to the stress with increased adrenaline. This action decreases dopamine in the brain. Now, dopamine is a neurotransmitter naturally produced in the body and is present in the regions of the brain that regulate movement, emotion, motivation, and the feeling of pleasure. This neurotransmitter also stabilizes brain activity *and regulates the flow of information* to other parts of the brain. So, if caffeine decreases dopamine, your thinking is not going to be any better.

Caffeine is also an addictive substance. That is why so many products have it listed in their ingredients panel. Manufacturers are not trying to make their product better by doing this. They toss it in there for one reason—to get you addicted so you will buy more of what they are selling. Pretty clever. Just think of all the other chemicals listed in ingredient panels of which we know nothing about. Why are they there? What are their side effects? What are they doing to our bodies?

Deception No. 2—Daylight saving time was sold by politicians as a harmless energy conservation measure.

The New England Journal of Medicine (Oct. 30, 2008) reported there were more heart attacks after daylight saving time was implemented. Why is that? Because when the brain that governs our sleep/awake rhythms is forced to move an hour forward or backward, an unneeded stress is placed on the body. You may have noticed this as you try to adjust to the time change each spring and fall. Our body's chemical, electrical, hormonal, and immunologic environments experience stress in adjusting to the change in rest patterns.

There are really few if any benefits from changing the time back and forth. This twice-a-year ritual increases stress and bumps up heart attack risk.

Why do we keep doing it? Perhaps stores want us to enjoy a longer shopping day. Perhaps we just want more daylight time to have fun. But we are paying a price for the pleasure.

Deception No. 3—Sugar is good for you.

This seems to be the message heralded by many food manufacturers. Look at the ingredients of most of your grocery store or fast-food favorites and you will find sugar or high fructose corn syrup—or under one of their many other names—listed as a major ingredient.

Someone once told me if we would tax corn syrup significantly, we would have no health crisis in this country because obesity levels would decline. But as long as sugar is relatively cheap, it will find its way into most foods.

There is another problem that's anything but sweet. Sugar is addictive. It acts on the brain to make you feel good. Think about it. How many times have you (and I) eaten an entire box of cookies instead of enjoying just one? Were we that hungry? No. After a while, receptors in our brains get used to sugar and it takes more and more of it to achieve the desired pleasure response. This is a classic example of an addiction under development.

Unfortunately, too many calories are also being consumed, leading to extra fat storage and the added stress extra weight brings to the system. We are being deceived into thinking there are no long-term consequences of eating an entire box of cookies—or chips, or candies, or whatever. Food manufacturers are blatantly and effectively addicting an entire generation. We were not designed to eat this way.

Deception No. 4—Bigger the better.

Supersize it! Doing so might achieve a short-term economic gain for a fast-food chain, but in the long run, we are all losers.

Here is a surprising fact. Long-term survival studies indicate the less we eat, the longer we live. Again, we need to think about how our actions of today will affect the future. We really need to be undersizing our food portions, unless our diets consist of high-nutrition, high-fiber, and whole-plant foods. Only then is it actually possible to eat more and weigh less. But if you eat the standard American diet, watch out. And do not let anyone—especially the fast-food industry—tell you different.

Deception No. 5—Cow's milk is good for you.

I'd have to say, of all the deceptions we face, this one leads the pack. Humans are the only mammals who continue to drink milk after the weaning period. And we are also the only mammal who drinks the milk of another species.

Epidemiologist T. Colin Campbell, in his book *The China Study*, provides compelling evidence milk is far from the healthy beverage advertisers say it is. As a matter of fact, after years of highly scientific research, he made this rather startling conclusion concerning the connection between milk consumption and cancer in tightly controlled laboratory animals:

"Casein, which makes up 87 percent of cow's milk protein, promoted all stages of the cancer process. What type of protein did not promote cancer, even at high levels of intake? The safe proteins were from plants, including wheat and soy." Then he adds, speaking of his now famous China study, "What made this project especially remarkable is that, among the many associations that are relevant to diet and disease, so many pointed to the same finding: people who ate the most animal-based foods got the most chronic disease. Even relatively small intakes of animal-based food were associated with adverse effects. People who ate the most plant-based foods were the healthiest and tended to avoid chronic disease" (pp. 6, 7).

Make no mistake about it. Milk is nothing more than liquid meat.

"But, what about calcium?" I hear you ask. Milk certainly contains calcium, placed there by the cow's body. We humans manufacture calcium as well. But here is the deception. When we drink cow's milk (or goat's milk), we are introducing an acidic food into our system because all animal-based foods are acidic. The body, which tries to maintain a balanced pH level that favors the alkaline side of the scale, immediately sets about attempting to neutralize this newly introduced acid. How does it do this? By applying its best neutralizer. And what is this all-important element that the body utilizes to tame the acid in the milk? It is the calcium stored in our bones. That's right. Milk does not build our bones. Instead, it causes the body to leach its own calcium into the blood stream in order to neutralize the intruder, thus actually *removing* calcium from the bones. Is it any wonder that in countries where the most milk is consumed, we find the greatest rate of osteoporosis?

Why don't we hear about this deception? Because the milk industry has taken a specific truth—milk contains calcium—and created a marketing scheme working to its advantage. We think we are doing something good for our bodies. But we are not. We are literally destroying the very bones the marketers say we are building.

I do not mean to gross you out, but if cow's could talk, what would you think if you saw one of those gentle creatures approaching a lactating woman and saying, "Excuse me, lady. I'm running a little short on milk. May I have some of yours to feed my calf?" In essence, that is exactly what we are doing to the cow. And although it has probably never been tested, I am pretty sure human milk would be just as unhealthy for the cow as cow's milk is for the human.

This situation leads us to our next deception.

Deception No. 6—The media tells the truth and wants the best for you.

The media can be a powerful tool for good. It can be a terrific vehicle for spreading the truth. I hope you believe this book is an example of that. But, think about it, the media is also all about making money for advertisers.

I have patients come to me with miracle substances they have read about in a magazine or discovered on the Internet. Some of these pills, potions, or procedures are harmless. But often well-meaning individuals spend a lot of money on substances that carry no evidence that they are truly beneficial. In fact, sometimes these magical potions do not even possess the ingredients they claim to contain. Remember, the Food and Drug Administration does not regulate many of these substances. Because of this, there is often no science behind the claims.

That is why I have created what I call the "Marcum Test" when it comes to such products. You might want to consider using such a process when you're facing a health product decision.

First, I ask myself, "Does this product make sense?" I know enough about the human body to realize most health problems require several responses, not just one. There is no "magic bullet" when it comes to building and maintaining optimum health. Anything claiming to cure a long list of ills does not get much of my attention. Yes, it may do one or two things well, but if it falls all over itself trying to convince you that you've just found the secret for all that ails you, keep looking.

Second, I want to know, "Is there science behind this?" I am not talking about a study created by the manufacturer of the product, which serves to prove its marketing claims. I am talking about hard scientific evidence supporting what the product says it can do.

And third, I ask myself, "Does this product or concept agree with the Owner's Manual, the Bible?" Where does it fit in with God's overall health plan for our lives?

Then, finally, I ask, "Is it available to all of God's creatures?" God is the ultimate unselfish being. He makes His "health products" available to all people everywhere. If what He created to keep us healthy is not naturally occurring someplace—or at least freely available at that location—we should not be living there. It is that simple.

Deception No. 7—We have a national health-care crisis.

I don't mean to sound unpatriotic, but no government has the solution to health care when 80 percent of disease in that nation or country is lifestyle-related. Can you see lawmakers in Washington, D.C., telling us how to live our lives? Wouldn't work. We would not listen. We are far too independent.

Our health-care crisis is not national. It is *personal*. And the answer has to come from within our own lives and the choices we make every day. Real change must be the result of sound education and clear-headed, unbiased thinking, not a majority vote.

Deception No. 8—Someone is protecting us.

With over 14,000 chemicals added to the American food supply on a regular basis, how can anyone be sure what these chemicals are doing to us and how they are reacting with other chemicals? The deception is that this practice is actually safe!

Many of these chemicals have absolutely no food value, and some are nothing more than addictive substances tossed in to boost sales. Consider these examples: Glutamate (MSG) and aspartame (an artificial sweetener) have been shown to be toxic to the neurons in young brains. Other food additives gaining attention include benzene (a colorless, volatile, flammable toxic liquid used in organic synthesis, as a solvent, *and as a motor fuel*), BHA (a phenolic—disinfectant—antioxidant used especially to preserve fats and oils in food), and anything hydrolyzed (the chemical process of decomposition). This stuff is in our food. In our food!

We do not understand how our bodies will react to these toxins. But if human history is any template, we are about to find out. We are all becoming laboratory rats in an ongoing study, the results of which I can guarantee will not be pretty.

That is what I love most about the whole foods God created for us to eat—no chemicals or additives necessary. No preservatives required. Not even a nutrition label needed. Whole foods straight from the hand of God are nutritious, delicious, and tailor-made for human consumption. No worries, no dangers, no deceptions.

Hey, I guess I was wrong. Someone *is* protecting us.

The Ripple Effect

Recently, Michelle came into my office suffering from chest pains. Why she was having chest pains is an example of what can happen when we deviate from God's original ideal for us—when we allow ourselves to live a deceived life. This is a story you will not soon forget.

For 20 years Michelle served an upscale company as an executive secretary. She told me every day she put on her high-heel shoes and happily headed off to work. Her shoes were expected office attire and reflected the company's image perfectly.

After 20 years her feet began to have significant problems. There was increasing pain each time she tried to walk, so she made an appointment with a podiatrist, who diagnosed the problem and recommended surgery. Because of the persistent pain, she stopped her regular exercise routine. Two operations later, she was still unable to walk comfortably, but found some relief from her infirmity in food. She quickly put on weight, which, in time, caused her to develop diabetes, hypertension, and sleep apnea. Her doctors placed her on medications and suggested a sleep mask. But Michelle still could not rest because of the severe pain in her feet so she started taking powerful narcotics and a sleeping pill. Subsequently she was replaced at work because her boss said she was not as sharp as she used to be.

The narcotics she was taking slowed down her bowels, and soon she had a bowel obstruction complicated by an infection. She was now also having chest pains, and that is why she came to see me.

When I heard her tale of woe, I just shook my head in amazement. What a horror story! When one stress to the body occurs—even if it occurs slowly—there is often a ripple effect. Michelle could have bypassed this entire cascade of illnesses if she had simply tossed her high-heel shoes in the dumpster 20 years ago and found a new job that allowed stylish flats.

When Michelle heard I was writing this book, she asked me to include her story, hoping to get people to think about the consequences of even the simplistic actions taken outside of God's design for our lives. The clothes we wear, the chemicals we smear on our bodies to smell or look good, the substances we ingest, the images we dwell on, the sounds we hear—all impact us in what can be dramatic ways. Like it or not, everything we do makes a difference—one way or another—to our health. I believe we owe it to ourselves to think about such things and not blindly follow popular or cultural trends. Doing so just might cause a ripple effect 20 years down the road. Trust me, when we live a life overrun by deceptions, there *will* be ripple effects.

But, if you have read this far, you know we have a standard with which to judge every decision we make. We know how we were designed to live. There is no mystery to solve or puzzle to piece together. God made us, understands perfectly what we need to do to stay healthy, and provides the needed elements each and every day of our lives. However, so few learn His principles of health and take advantage of His guidance.

What happened to change our world so profoundly? How did we get from the Garden of Eden to the mess we now call life? The answers to those two questions will form the very foundation of healthy living for you and your family. In the story of earth's most horrible deception, we find both the causes of all disease, and the cures for all infirmities. It is also where we will discover the incredible power and eternal benefits of the heart of health.

Chapter 15

The Lie

O n a blustery cold January morning in 2007, a man made his way to the Metro Station in Washington, D.C., and took up a position in the bustling lobby. With streams of people passing by, he retrieved a violin from the case he was carrying and began to adeptly tune the strings. Once satisfied the tones would be perfect and the bow was adjusted properly, he lifted the instrument to his chin and began to play.

The notes he created mingled with the shuffling of shoes, clanking of coins being dropped into ticket machines, clatter of the turnstiles, and distant rumble of the trains. For 45 minutes he filled the busy enclosure with intricate trills and the metered melodies of Johann Sebastian Bach, never missing a note. His inflections and emotional renderings were flawless.

While he played, one middle-aged man stopped for a moment, and then moved on. A few minutes later, a woman tossed a dollar bill into the open violin case as she hurried by. Several children paused quizzically before being dragged away by preoccupied parents.

After completing his 45-minute concert, the man counted up his earnings for the morning. He found $32 in his case, placed there by approximately 20 people, none of whom had stopped to listen. As a matter of fact, no one—save the middle-aged man—had taken the time to enjoy the music.

No one had applauded or shown more than a passing interest in the musician. What they did not know—or even try to discover—was that the man in the lobby was Joshua Bell, one of the world's greatest violinists. The instrument he was playing was valued at more than $3.5 million dollars. Just two days before, this same musician had performed in Boston to a packed concert hall where seats averaged $100 each.

It is evident by this story that, at such an unusual time and in such an unusual place, several thousand individuals failed to recognize one of the most talented musicians of our generation playing some of the finest music ever written on one of the most beautiful instruments ever created. They simply did not stop to listen.

Is this happening to you? Are you too busy, too preoccupied, too overcome with the realities of living on this deceived planet to listen to your Creator talking to you about your health—perhaps at times and places where you would least expect it? If the answer is yes, there is a reason. And that reason took root in a garden many years ago.

Voice in the Tree

Much had already taken place in the universe before Adam and Eve began walking the paths of their beautiful garden. According to Scripture, one of God's most talented and wise creations, an angel named Lucifer, became disenchanted with how things were. Bible scholars agree this special being felt he was not being given the attention he deserved, so he started a rumor campaign against God, telling the other created beings how he—and they—were nothing more than subjects under the thumb of a heartless dictator.

To make a long story short, this Lucifer, who was also called the "dragon" in the Bible, finally gained enough followers, and stirred up enough trouble, God—also called "Michael" in Scripture—felt compelled to take action. Here is how John the revelator described what happened next: "And there was war in heaven. Michael and his angels fought against the dragon, and the dragon and his angels fought back. But he was not strong enough, and they lost their place in heaven. The great dragon was hurled down—that ancient serpent called the devil, or Satan, who leads the whole world astray. He was hurled to the earth, and his angels with him" (Revelation 12:7-9).

Referring to this event—and Satan's eventual destruction—as well as providing a tiny glimpse into the motivation behind Satan's rebellion, the Old Testament prophet Isaiah writes: "How you have fallen from heaven, O morning star, son of the dawn! You have been cast down to the earth, you who once laid low the nations! You said in your heart, 'I will ascend to heaven; I will raise my throne above the stars of God; I will sit enthroned on the mount of assembly, on the utmost heights of the sacred mountain. I will ascend above the tops of the clouds; I will make myself like the Most High.' But you are brought down to the grave, to the depths of the pit" (Isaiah 14:12-15).

Satan sure used the word "I" a lot, didn't he? He was all about what *he* wanted, what *he* was trying to accomplish, what made *him* feel good about himself. You might even call him selfish. God, on the other hand, is all about others, about you . . . and me. He is focused on us, on *our* well-being. Is it any wonder such two opposing factions could not coexist within the perfect harmony of heaven?

So, Satan loses his exalted position in the presence of God and ends up in the only place in the universe where he would not be immediately expelled by the inhabitants—our brand-new, virtually unpopulated earth. And Eve found him one day, appearing in the form of a beautiful, winged serpent draped lazily among the branches of a tree.

We pick up the story in Genesis, chapter 3, starting with verse 1: "Now the serpent was more crafty than any of the wild animals the Lord God had made. He said to the woman, 'Did God really say, "You must not eat from any tree in the garden"?'"

First of all, we must remember God had, indeed, conversed with Adam concerning the very tree in which the serpent now sprawled. He told him, "You are free to eat from any tree in the garden; but you must not eat from the tree of the knowledge of good and evil, for when you eat of it you will surely die" (Genesis 2:16, 17).

Eve must have been aware of this command because she calmly answered the serpent, "We may eat fruit from the trees in the garden, but God did say, 'You must not eat fruit from the tree that is in the middle of the garden, and you must not touch it, or you will die'" (Genesis 3:2, 3). This word "die" must have been a foreign concept to them.

What happened next is still impacting our lives today. The words Satan spoke in response to Eve's statement form the very core of our present health crises, our spiritual detachments, our relationship struggles, and our many mental diseases. Lowering himself to eye level with the woman, the serpent smiled reassuringly and said in a soothing, confident voice, "You will not surely die. . . . For God knows that when you eat of it your eyes will be opened, and you will be like God, knowing good and evil" (verses 4, 5).

You will not surely die. Go ahead. Eat the forbidden fruit, choose whatever you want, enjoy all the junk food your heart desires, completely ignore your circadian rhythm, fill your mind with scenes of depravity and violence, stare at a computer terminal all day, text instead of talking, ride instead of walking, lust instead of loving, worship technology, sports, and anything else except the true God; it won't hurt you. What does God know? He is a heartless dictator who just wants you to be His slave and do exactly what He says or . . . well . . . look what happened to me. I got tossed from heaven because I dared confront Him with the truth.

"You will not surely die." Millions of people still believe these words when they light up their first cigarette, fill their stomachs with what satisfies their addictive-perverted taste buds, hurry past nutrition-packed foods in the grocery store as they pile their shopping carts high with highly processed favorites. How many people shuffle off to the doctor's office seeking answers to their illnesses when, like Eve, the garden in which they live overflows with what they really need to build and maintain optimum health?

The same serpent that slithered among the branches of that long-forgotten tree still moves in the shadows of our lives today, ready to repeat his deadly declaration in our times of indecision. "You will not surely die."

God's words to Adam and Eve were more than a warning. They were identifying a set of laws—the very same laws holding the universe in place. His revelation also identified, in no uncertain terms, what would happen if those laws were broken. Death, and the self-imposed sicknesses that often result in death, is not a punishment from God. The fact Adam and Eve—and every generation to this moment—have passed away is not because God is punishing anyone for breaking His laws. You jump out of an airplane without a parachute and you die, not because God is unhappy with you, but because breaking certain laws brings about certain consequences. When God told Adam if he ate of the forbidden fruit, he would die, He was not bringing judgment down on the man's head. He was simply allowing earth's first humans to make a choice based on complete and proper information. Don't eat, you live forever. Eat, you die. Period.

When He spoke to Adam, the Creator was identifying two paths to follow—one based on universal law, the other based on life lived outside that law. The latter is where Satan had chosen to spend his existence. In essence, God was saying, "Adam, Eve, here's the deal. My laws, based on love and liberty, will lead to eternal life. You can walk with Me, talk face-to-face with Me, and enjoy all the benefits of living your life in harmony with My universal laws. But, I'm no dictator. I know love without liberty is not love at all. So I give you the ability to choose. You can determine your own future. You can decide which path you want to follow. The tree of which I am speaking represents everything that is not within My path. I put it there so you can demonstrate to Me—and all created beings—you *choose* to remain loyal to My laws of love. You have got to understand by eating the fruit of that tree, you will be switching paths, and the consequence of doing so will mean eternal separation from Me. You . . . will . . . die."

The power of choice—the most amazing and dangerous gift God ever bestowed on humankind—is a product of love, not dominion.

Christian psychiatrist and author Dr. Timothy Jennings puts it this way in his book, *Could It Be This Simple?*: "It is impossible for love to exist in an atmosphere without freedom. If you're not sure, try it on your spouse. Tell him or her that if they don't love you, you will kill them. Restrict your spouse's liberties, and see what happens to love. The law of liberty is one of the cornerstone principles of God's government. As God is love, He necessarily *must* respect the liberty and individuality of His intelligent creatures. To do otherwise would destroy love and incite rebellion" (p. 48).

It was safely within this very liberty that Eve walked in the garden that day. It was because of this liberty the serpent was able to spew his verbal venom on such an innocent woman. And it was within the boundaries set forth by liberty that Eve did the unthinkable. "When the woman saw that the fruit of the tree was good for food and pleasing to the eye, and also desirable for gaining wisdom, she took some and ate it. She also gave some to her husband, who was with her, and he ate it" (Genesis 3:6).

Later in the Old Testament, King Solomon stated what, by then, was totally obvious to everyone. "There is a way that seems right to a man, but in the end it leads to death" (Proverbs 14:12).

Two paths—one comfortably within God's law of love; the other outside that law. Two results—one future designed by the loving mind of a Creator God; the other constructed by a mind filled with rebellion and self-interest. Adam and Eve chose the second path, and we are still stumbling along its rugged and dangerous outline today. This second path has led to deceptions, causing stress on the system including our very own DNA, and the resultant change in chemistry. This then leads to symptoms and a need for modern medicine.

But—and here is the best news any cardiologist or health practitioner can give to a patient—the first path still exists! The laws that govern it, shape it, and determine its destination still wait for anyone who chooses to turn his or her back on the deceptions perpetuated by Satan and his empire. It is *only* along this path optimum health can be found. *Only* on the path created by love do we find the answers to our most troubling health questions. Contrary to what Satan has been saying for thousands of years, it is *only* on this path we can find the whole, unblemished truth about how to overcome disease and—just as important—reestablish our lost connection with the God who created us.

Eden set the standard for gaining and maintaining optimal physical health. Within those seven days of Creation, we discovered the powerful laws governing the well-being of every creature on earth. But there was another element to Satan's statement to Eve that is just as destructive to minds and bodies as the belief that God's laws weren't really put in place for our ultimate good. If you read between the lines, you uncover a frightening undercurrent in which many struggle to this day. What so few realize is this undercurrent—this hidden message—or shall we say deception can make you very, very sick.

Chapter 16

The Path of Truth

I n his fascinating book *Cheating Death* Dr. Sanjay Gupta, a neurosurgeon, deftly describes many situations in which the end of life is delayed or completely avoided—at least for the time being. Dr. Gupta, who has been described as "The World's Doctor," brings to light many instances in which technology has evolved to the point where it can actually, in his words, "cheat death." This amazing technology includes utilizing the effects of hypothermia, applying innovative resuscitation techniques, using elements such as hydrogen sulfide to help trauma victims, and performing delicate in utero procedures correcting birth defects, urinary blockages, and diaphragmatic hernias.

This new technology is "buying time" to enable further healing either through modern medicine or allowing the body to ultimately repair what is wrong.

While we mere mortals cannot understand all aspects of healing, God has given us the intelligence to apply His powerful laws of health even though at times we may not fully comprehend how these laws operate. The God who made us is truly at the center of every healing encounter and should be a part of every treatment plan. The One who makes it all possible should lead modern medicine. The only way "to cheat death" is to utilize God's Health Plan. Remember, death was not part of the plan, but a result of a path chosen.

Which brings up the next question: In the midst of the worldwide health crisis, why are we not hearing more about God's original Health Plan? People like David need surgeries, medications, and are sicker than ever before. There is real suffering all around. One would think something needs to change, the sooner the better. We in the healing world are missing something. Why are we not looking for something new, a new approach? Why are we not looking at the real cause of the problem?

I must admit modern technology is exciting, and the ability to "cheat" death is dramatic. I enjoy the medical dramas too, but why are we not talking about the Master Healer as the leader of the health-care team? Why have we moved so far from the original plan? Why? Why? Why? If we understand "why" this has happened to our world, perhaps we can rediscover the balance in healing.

I think it is high time to, as Paul Harvey used to say, hear "the rest of the story." The rest of the story will answer the question "Why." Just as there is a cause for illness, there is a reason that we are searching for healing in all the wrong places. There is a deception taking place of which many are unaware.

Deeper Antagonism

I believe the answer to why is based on the deception found in the Garden of Eden where a beautiful serpent hung from the branches and spoke to Eve one day. As we have discovered, his words originated from a heart darkened by self-interest and rebellion. He not only insisted that God was not telling the truth; he revealed a deeper antagonism for the Creator. In a voice soothing yet provoking, Satan inferred that God was misrepresenting Himself. There was no love in Satan's actions. The true nature of God was being challenged. Who would want a God like this to be in charge of healing?

I like the illustration my colleague, Christian psychiatrist Dr. Timothy Jennings, shares with many of his patients when discussing the subject of love and trust. He asks them to consider this scenario: Someone you know says your spouse has been cheating on you. He or she even presents false evidence. How do you feel about your spouse after that information is shared? The fact your husband or wife is totally innocent of any wrongdoing means nothing *if you believe the lie*. And, if you believe the lie, does your relationship change? Do you find it hard to trust your spouse? Do you believe anything he or she says from that moment on?

Then Dr. Jennings drives the story home with these words: "Lies believed break the circle of love and trust. This leads to a spirit of fear, selfishness, and rebellion."

Sound familiar? I think it is safe to say Satan ran a highly successful rumor campaign against God. His lie—God is an enslaving dictator with little regard for the "little people" in His heavenly kingdom—convinced many angels to rebel, even though there was no truth in the argument. Why do I bring this up? Unless we understand the real problem and its origin, we do not have a chance at finding the solution. This original deception—God can't be trusted—and the subsequent lies about His character were the real problem. This set up a cascade of events we are still a part of today.

Later this same deceiver faces Adam and Eve in the garden, and from his mouth issues more venom. "You will not surely die" was a statement meant to cast doubt on God's honesty and integrity. "You can cheat death." Then he added this devastating punch line. "For God knows that when you eat of it your eyes will be opened, and you will be like God, knowing good and evil" (Genesis 3:5).

The serpent was right—to a point. Having disobeyed a direct command from God—don't eat from that tree—Adam's and Eve's eyes were certainly now open to knowing good and evil. They had known good, but now they knew for the first time the unsettling discomfort of doing evil.

It is the statement "you will be like God" that caused the most devastating rift between the Creator and His two freshly minted humans. Suddenly, in their minds, God was not this perfect being filled with unselfish love and wisdom. If they were now "like God," that meant He must be flawed, self-seeking, and prone to doubt, just as they were now feeling inside. In other words, God's character had been transformed in their minds. Because they had believed a lie and disobeyed, the circle of love and trust was broken and their precious Creator and friend was now someone they did not trust. Very quickly, that mistrust turned to fear. The deception was taking root and beginning to grow. Why should we believe the health plan or anything this type of God recommends?

False God

In his book *The Sign,* Shawn Boonstra, speaker/director of It Is Written International Television, writes: "If human beings—created in the image of God—routinely violate God's moral principles, it discredits the idea that His requirements are reasonable or that obeying them is even *possible.* It casts a shadow of doubt over the viability of God's government." What does this statement mean? As we fall into deceptions we gradually become enslaved in them. The devil reiterates, "I *told* you there was something wrong with God's way! *No one* can live up to His expectations!" This is exactly where Adam and Eve unfortunately found themselves, and we wonder why God's Health Plan is not getting any attention.

"But, Doctor Marcum," I hear you saying, "I do not believe Satan's lies about God!"

I am so thankful for every person who claims this, because this means he or she is truly trying to serve the God they love. But, then I must ask a very pointed and, in some circles, highly controversial question: "Is the God you love and worship the true God, or one based on lies—falsehoods of which you may not even be aware? Are you worshipping God or a 'being' society has created?" Think about this for a few minutes. This is important. Allow me to provide some examples of this horrible deception.

Many Christians worship a God who, in essence, says, "I love you so much. I created the world for you and died on the cross for you, and will someday come and take you home to live with Me in heaven forever and ever. However, if you break My commandments or turn your back on My love, I will kill you."

Think long and hard about what I just said. Is that your God? Believing in such a "hell and brimstone" heavenly Father might provide a good motivation for obedience, but it hardly creates a comfortable foundation to build a loving relationship.

There's more. Continuing our Genesis story, we read what happened after Adam and Eve's encounter with the serpent: "Then the man and his wife heard the sound of the Lord God as he was walking in the garden in the cool of the day, and they hid from the Lord God among the trees of the garden. But the Lord God called to the man, 'Where are you?'

"He answered, 'I heard you in the garden, and I was afraid'" (Genesis 3:8-10).

Afraid? Of God? Why?

"I was afraid because I was naked; so I hid.'

"And [the Lord] said, 'Who told you that you were naked? Have you eaten from the tree that I commanded you not to eat from?'" (verses 10, 11).

There's something interesting here. Adam had apparently been stripped of the divine glory that "clothed" both him and Eve, a covering allowing them to feel completely at ease in the presence of their Creator. They were now uncomfortable. This was not part of the original plan. Once again I am reminded of Dr. Jennings' words: "Lies believed break the circle of love and trust, leading to a spirit of fear, selfishness, and rebellion."

Then God asked Adam, "Who told you that you were naked?" (verse 11).

Wait a minute! It seems that God was not the force generating the grinding guilt creating Adam's fear. Adam and Eve felt guilty—and naked—even before the Lord showed up. I believe they were feeling the uncertainty and dread generated from walking the path prepared by Satan. They were now off course. Something was far from right. For the first time they were experiencing the stress originating from living outside the protective presence of their Creator. Their chemistry was changing—and not for the good. They had placed themselves firmly on the wrong path—the path that, according to God, leads to death.

Notice that this death is a result of deception, not an act of God. Our heavenly Father lovingly grants us the freedom to walk down the path that separates us from Him and reap the results of our actions.

When Adam and Eve discovered the Lord was nearby looking for them, they hid in the bushes. After all, the God who made them must be a vengeful God. Didn't He throw Satan and his followers out of heaven simply because they dared to disagree with Him?

Do you see the transformation taking place here? God had done no wrong, but Adam and Eve believed Satan's lies, and lies believed change everything. Are we running and hiding from our true healer? Does it make any sense to run from love? Has the world told us how to think of and relate to God? Has an accurate picture been portrayed or another deception been introduced?

The Woman

Let's spend a moment in the New Testament exploring another popular misconception of our heavenly Father. We find a revealing story in the book of John, chapter 8. A group of self-righteous and very "religious" men come before Jesus dragging with them a woman "caught in the act of adultery." "Teacher," they say, shoving their victim down at Christ's feet, "in the Law Moses commanded us to stone such women. Now what do you say" (verses 4, 5)?

According to John's account, Jesus "bent down and started to write on the ground with his finger. When they kept on questioning him, he straightened up and said to them, 'If any one of you is without sin, let him be the first to throw a stone at her'" (verses 6, 7).

I am not sure what He wrote on the ground—perhaps street addresses or people's names—but whatever information He scratched in the dirt made an impression because, one by one, the accusers decided they had important appointments elsewhere. Finally, only Jesus and the woman remained.

Listen carefully to what Jesus says next and see if this matches your concept of the God you worship. "Jesus straightened up and asked her, 'Woman, where are they? Has no one condemned you?'

"'No one, sir,' she said.

"'Then neither do I condemn you,' Jesus declared. 'Go now and leave your life of sin'" (verses 10, 11).

According to this story, the worthlessness we feel when we have sinned, when we have been deceived, is not from God. Here was a woman caught in the very act of adultery. There was no question she was not living the plan set up at Creation. But Christ—who was fully aware of this—said He did not condemn her. He basically told her, "What you were doing is wrong and not good for you, so stop doing it!" No judgment, no dire warning of impending punishment, no thunderous sermons about hellfire, no unyielding demand for repentance, no condemnation. But, you know what? I have a feeling that woman, fresh from the arms of a married man who was not her husband, found something unexpected that day. She discovered a type of love that can turn fearful sinners into thankful, adoring worshippers. She found, at the feet of Jesus, an acceptance that no church, no society, no culture offered her. She, perhaps for the first time, caught a glimpse of the real God, the true God from whom humankind had been hiding since Adam and Eve ate the fruit from the forbidden tree; since they switched paths from God's way to Satan's way and took the whole world with them. She, like so many of us, had believed a lie. Now she was looking directly into the face of absolute truth, and it transformed her life forever. Her chemistry was changing. Healing had begun.

"Yeah, well, when you are dealing with Jesus, that is one thing. But God the Father, watch out! He's the judge, jury, and executioner all rolled into one."

Really? Listen to what Jesus said when one of His disciples asked Him a very direct question during what Christians call "The Last Supper."

Christ has just made the statement "No one comes to the Father except through me." This was followed by "If you really knew me, you would know my Father as well. From now on, you do know him and have seen him" (John 14:6, 7).

Here is what happened next: "Philip said, 'Lord, show us the Father and that will be enough for us.'

"Jesus answered: 'Don't you know me, Philip, even after I have been among you such a long time? Anyone who has seen me has seen the Father. How can you say, "Show us the Father"? Don't you believe that I am in the Father, and that the Father is in me? The words I say to you are not just my own. Rather, it is the Father, living in me, who is doing his work'" (verses 8-10). God was dispelling the deceptions and showing the truth, what love looked like through His Son. This was His character. He was not at all like the portrait painted by Satan. Here was proof.

If I were to ask you, "Who would you rather spend the rest of eternity with, Jesus or God the Father?" I have a feeling many would say, "Give me Jesus!" Why? Because so many of us think God the Father is a harsh, demanding judge with whom Jesus is pleading our case, asking for leniency. Where did *that* come from?

It came from Eden. It came from the branches of the tree of the knowledge of good and evil. It came from the mouth of the master deceiver, Satan. Jesus and His Father are one in thought, one in action, and one in their determination to bring saving love into every life. They long to heal. The reason we are not being drawn to God as the Master Healer, the Great Physician, and His Health Plan is the lies and deceptions passed down from generation to generation.

Apart From God

I could go on and on, but I won't. There are many resources available to help you on this journey to a clearer and more realistic picture of our heavenly Father. But I have brought you here for a reason. We're trying to discover why we have departed from the original health plan given at Creation. Simply put, we've been deceived regarding the nature of God and now we fear Him instead of loving Him. Since Eden, the misconceptions about God have driven us further and further apart from the God who made us. We've been traveling down the slippery slopes of self-worship and a dependence on our own intelligence to right our wrongs, bring meaning to our lives, and heal our bodies. We've been carried here on the wings of the greatest deception of all—that God really is not our friend, our guide, and our hope. And when we lose hope, when we feel alone in this world, when we harbor an unspoken fear of the God of the universe, we introduce stress into our bodies. We change the chemistry that keeps us healthy.

We were designed to worship and love the true God, the God of love. When this does not occur, we're driven onto the path of destructive habits and empty relationships. Each of these conditions eats away at our mind, body, and spirit like a cancer eats away muscle, bone, and flesh.

But, there is a medicine—an antidote for this condition. I have seen it work time and time again. It is available to all people everywhere, and it does not cost a penny. You just have to know where to find it.

Chapter 17

The Heart of Health

David looked at me through questioning eyes. "So I can do anything I want and God will still love me?"

I thought for a moment before I responded. "The answer to your question is . . . yes. God is in the loving business," I said. "He is all about life, not death."

My patient had made a remarkable recovery from his heart attack. For months now, he had been doing his best to follow the health guidelines revealed in our Owner's Manual, the Bible. He was learning to enjoy whole food—foods as grown—and had traded his daily sugar-filled soda pops for glasses of pure, refreshing water. He began walking with his supportive wife each day, said good-bye to late-night television so he could get more sleep, and even started resting one day a week. David was feeling great, looking amazing—compared to when we first met—and admitted he had more energy than ever. I noticed on his chart his weight was dropping and cheered with him when test results revealed no new plaque was building up in his arteries. He was experiencing firsthand the incredible power of God's Health Plan.

But I also knew there was more to gaining optimum health than doing all the right things physically. The body and mind are connected in very powerful ways, and a stressed mind can alter the body's chemistry just as a stressed body can wreck havoc on the mind. If I wanted David to experience even better health, I needed to make sure there was nothing causing undue tension on his *brain*. This is one area of recovery many physicians miss or simply ignore.

"David," I explained, "stress can originate from brains damaged by misconceptions concerning God. Let me explain."

There are definitely evil forces among us—real evil that is destructive and deadly. This evil leads to deception, which in turn takes us away from God's plan—the original source of health. I picked up my Bible and thumbed through the pages. "For the wages of sin is death" (Romans 6:23). Deception and sin don't need a judge to bring negative consequences to those who travel on this path.

I think we can all agree there is definitely sin in this world. But did you notice something interesting here? The apostle Paul, the writer of Romans, describes death as a "wage" of sin. A wage is not a penalty. A wage is payment for services rendered. If you go against God's law, you are eventually paid with death. Then the text continues: "But the gift of God is eternal life in Christ Jesus our Lord." This passage identifies those two paths I talked about earlier—Satan's path and God's path. It also reveals just where those two paths lead—one to life, one to death. So, if you happen to be walking along Satan's path toward death and you end up dead, did God just zap you with a punishment, or did you simply reach your chosen destination?

As I have said before, the path of deception is self-destructive. It does a very thorough job of ruining lives, breaking hearts, and raining down hurt and agony on those who choose to follow this path. I guess you could say this path is self-judging. It is its own prosecutor and executioner as well.

"Before you had your heart attack, were you on this path, David?" I asked my patient.

David frowned. "Do you think I was being deceived and on the wrong path?"

I smiled. "David, I'm calling you a stumbler who fell along the path. Welcome to the club. According to the Bible, we are all sinners living in a sinful world. But God's path runs right through this sinful planet. It is available for any foot to follow. I am happy to say, even though you stumbled, that's the path you are walking on right now. How does it feel?"

David grinned shyly. "Feels great."

"You see," I continued, "while you were walking on the old path, you broke some very important health laws. You ate huge amounts of nutritionally-void junk food, lived a sedentary life, and allowed the stresses of everyday living to overpower you. So, was your heart attack a judgment from God? No. It was the result of breaking those health laws.

"Now, I tell you this because many people believe God is a stern judge just waiting to see us fail so He can pronounce judgment on us. This type of belief stresses the brain. An attitude like this not only separates us even further from our heavenly Father; it totally affects our health."

Rearview Mirror

"Have you ever been driving in your car and suddenly noticed in your rearview mirror a police officer following you? At that moment, if you're like me, you become the best driver on earth. You nail the speed limit, use your turn signals appropriately, and keep your tires between the lines like never before. Why do you do that?"

David chuckled. "I don't want to get caught breaking the law."

"Are you feeling relaxed, happy, contented?"

"No way! I'm feeling tense."

"Even though you are doing everything right?"

"Well . . . yeah!"

"OK. And let's say you make a turn, and the police officer follows you. You make another turn, and the cop car remains on your tail. How are you feeling now?"

David laughed. "Let's just say I'm trying to figure out if my registration is up to date, whether my license has expired, whether I have any unpaid parking tickets, and if my insurance check was mailed in on time last month. In other words, I'm stressed."

"So," I pressed, "you're doing absolutely nothing wrong, yet you are completely stressed out over what the cop is doing back there and what he might think of you—or know about you?"

My patient nodded. "Yup. That's about right."

"David," I said, "that is how many people feel about God. He is back there, following them, ready to pounce, ready to condemn, ready to toss them straight into hell. They live their lives in stress and worry. More to the point, they live their life in fear—fear of the one source who can bring true healing to their mind, body, and spirit. Satan knows as long as you live in fear, you cannot enjoy optimum health. That is why he planted his unfair, untrue, and totally unsubstantiated image of God in Adam's and Eve's minds. He understood that fear is an incredibly powerful stressor, even capable of undoing the other good things we do for ourselves.

"Fear has many names—worry, guilt, uncertainty, anger. As long as we fail to grasp the true nature and character of God, our hearts will harbor hidden fear. This is not healthy, nor was this part of the original plan. When the mind is stressed, the body follows this lead chemically.

"But, God is not the condemning judge Satan wants us to believe He is.

He's something far different."

David leaned forward in his chair. "So, what is He?"

"Do you know who Lance Armstrong is?"

My patient blinked. "God is a world-class bicycle racer?"

I grinned and continued. "When Lance Armstrong races in a tournament, what does he usually have following him?"

"All the other racers?"

"Well, yes, but I am thinking about the van."

"The van?"

"There is always this van following him wherever he goes."

David smiled. "Oh, you mean his support team."

"That's right. And, are the people in the car there to record his mistakes, criticize his judgment, and make him feel bad when he does something wrong?"

"No," David interrupted. "They are there to help him fix his bicycle if it breaks, offer assistance if he's injured in a crash, and shout encouragement."

"That's right," I said. "You see, David, God is like the van. He is following us through life not to condemn, but to help. He knows we will need help when we are deceived and sin. And, here is what is really amazing about this whole thing. God faithfully follows us no matter which of the two paths we happen to be on."

My patient sat in silence for a long moment. I could see the wheels turning in his mind as thoughts he had never entertained sprang to life. He was beginning to see the true face of God. He was beginning to encounter, like the woman at Christ's feet, the heart of health.

"David," I continued, "the same God who created laws to help us build and maintain optimum physical health also set in place laws allowing our brains— our thoughts—to become healthy as well. Those laws are tied directly into how we perceive God. As long as we fear Him—like we fear the police officer following us—we can never enjoy optimum health of mind *or* body. It is just not possible, because the mind has so much influence over the body.

"And if we are afraid of Him, we are a lot less willing to believe Him. Suddenly, those health laws He set in place in Eden become nothing more than outdated ancient rituals with little or no relevance to us today. We turn from the Creator to our own understanding or to modern medical practices as our go-to source for health information and guidance. This places us firmly on the wrong path, and we begin a journey leading in the wrong direction. God does not condemn us for our choices. But we are making it very, very hard for Him to get through to us with the truth. However, He never quits trying. He is always following in the van."

I studied my patient carefully. "When you go to the store, walk the halls of your office building, or even sit in church, what do you see? Do you see healthy people who are managing their weight correctly, controlling their blood sugar and blood pressure, and taking the moral high ground in life? Or do you see people lost in confusion, desperately depending on the latest wonder drug or high-tech procedure to bring quality back into their lives?"

David thought for a moment. "It does not look very good out there, Doc," he admitted.

"That is because so many need the medicine I am about to share with you—a medicine so powerful, so overwhelming that sickness and disease, anger and resentment, fear and uncertainty cannot survive for long in its presence. It is hands down the most amazing antidote available on this earth. Would you like to know what it is?"

My patient nodded. "Doctor Marcum, I really want to know. Bring it on!"

Window of Opportunity

The time had come. The moment was right. My patient David had opened the door, and I was ready to share what I had learned.

Making people whole again after they have experienced a heart attack depends on several factors: the amount of damage done to the heart by the attack, the body's response to the various medicines and procedures introduced, the patient's willingness to follow instructions given by his or her cardiologist and recovery team, and just how serious the patient is about regaining health once the acute stage has passed. The damage to David's heart was minimal, owing to the fact that when the attack reached a climax he was talking to a cardiologist. Most people are not that fortunate.

When it comes to heart attacks, timing is everything. The window of opportunity for receiving lifesaving help is not measured in days. It is measured in minutes—sometimes seconds. David was very, very fortunate.

There is another window of opportunity that opens for a short period of time once the patient is out of danger and back home again. He or she has been frightened by their experience and is willing to make some changes. It is during these few short months—sometimes even weeks—that I try to make my case concerning the true source of health.

Far too many times I have observed patients stumbling across my threshold—people, like David, whom the health-care team has brought back from the very brink of death, who return with the same health problems recurring again and again. Why? They did not address the cause of the original problem. They did not change their lifestyle to accommodate their altered condition. Believe me, if you have survived bypass surgery, you've been altered.

As I said before, nothing is "fixed" by the experience. You've simply been handed a second chance, and I thank God for the science behind our ability to accomplish that. But, so many patients simply go back to the same old foods, the same old bad habits, the same old worries and anxieties, and the same old lack of desire to do the sometimes hard work necessary to keep them healthy. They do not want to change their lives. They just want me to make them strong enough so they can go back to living as before.

Pharmaceutical companies depend heavily on this type of patient. The last thing they want this man or woman to do is die . . . or get well. Unfortunately, some medical professionals march under the same banner.

But God calls us to be healers—all of us—and that includes me. He wants us to come back to the "original health plan." And if I know the true source of healing, I am going to share the information, even if doing so puts a dent in some drug company's bottom line.

One More Chance

Just before His betrayal and crucifixion, Jesus was enjoying a final meal with His precious disciples. He had just sent Judas away and was now left with 11 followers in the upper room. Christ understood He had only one more chance at getting through to these men before the storm of His arrest, mock trial, and execution swept through their lives.

Summoning their attention, He called out, "A new commandment I give you" (John 13:34). The disciples, as Jews, understood and obeyed the Ten Commandments, which had been handed down at Sinai to their ancestors— rules and regulations that would forever identify them as children of the one true God. But now Christ was facing a very different situation than He faced with ex-slave Moses, fresh out of Egyptian bondage. He was now talking to "modern" men, well versed in the how-to of their ancient faith. From this moment on, each disciple would need something more than a set of rules to follow. He knew very soon they would need something much more than a set of rules in their service to the world.

"A new commandment I give you," Christ continued. "Love one another. As I have loved you, so you must love one another." This was the voice of God speaking.

Knowing and obeying a set of rules and regulations would no longer be enough. Doing good was not enough. Preaching well was not enough. These 11 men needed something more. They needed to love.

This concept was not new in Christ's ministry. When the rich young ruler mentioned in Luke 18 came to see Jesus with the question "What must I do to inherit eternal life?" Christ, at first, took the traditional line. "You know the commandments," He said. "Do not commit adultery, do not murder, do not steal, do not give false testimony, honor your father and mother" (verses 18-20).

The ruler nodded. "All these I have kept since I was a boy," he stated.

Then Jesus added the most important, missing element. "You still lack one thing," He told His visitor. "Sell everything you have and give to the poor, and you will have treasure in heaven. Then come, follow me" (verses 21, 22). Become unselfish. Love.

The reaction of the ruler spoke volumes. "When he heard this, he became very sad, because he was a man of great wealth" (verse 23).

What the rich young ruler lacked was love—love for those without riches, love for those who did not have the opportunities he enjoyed, love for the "little people" who swarmed about him day in and day out. Who or what did he really worship? While being rich is certainly no sin, making money and the accumulation of things the determining factor for every decision you make certainly opens the door to selfishness and greed.

But, why love? Why is it so important? What did Christ know about it?

I am not an ordained minister. I have not studied at the best schools of religion or delved deeply into the ancient texts and the spiritual writings filling the libraries of theological seminaries.

But I do know a thing or two about medicine and the human body. As I have studied health in general and the heart in particular, I have discovered something incredible. Love is a healing force. It can often accomplish what medicine, procedures, or natural remedies cannot. I have seen it in action far too many times to dismiss it simply as an emotion. And I am not just talking about *being* loved. I am talking about maintaining a loving attitude and *giving* love.

What Is Love?

How do we define such an important concept as love? Some say, "It is putting someone else's interest before your own." "God is love," others insist. But I have got my own illustration that defines—in a small part—what love means to me.

When I come home from a long session at work, no matter what the hour or what worries may be weighing on my mind, my two dogs, Max and Daphne, greet me at the door. You would think they had not seen me for months! They are simply beside themselves with joy and eagerly follow me around just waiting for me to respond to their overflow of emotions. Those with pets can certainly relate to this. Even if when I left that morning I had punished them for something they'd done like mess on the floor or gnaw a hole in the furniture, all is forgotten in their unrestrained joy at my return.

You know what? The sight of those two little dogs eagerly waiting for me at the door does something to me deep inside. For a moment at least, the worries crowding my mind vanish. My weariness fades. My facial muscles automatically pull my lips into a happy smile. From an emotional standpoint, I am feeling pretty good. But I also know that throughout my body chemical changes are taking place bringing health and healing to every cell. That's right. My dogs are helping to bring healing to my heart, my bones, my organs, and my blood—all of me. Their unconditional, no-holds-barred love lowers my stress levels, decreases my heart rate, dilates my blood vessels, and relaxes my mind in ways no single medication can boast.

I must hasten to add seeing my two children at the door or catching a glimpse of my beautiful wife walking down the hall does the same thing. Love is an unbelievably powerful prescription.

It is overpowering. It bypasses stress and worry and injects incredible amounts of healing energies into the human body. Tests using very sophisticated devices have recorded its profound effect on the mind, body, and spirit of countless individuals. It is no surprise to me when people say, "The moment I fell in love, the sky was bluer, the grass was greener, and even the air smelled wonderful." If they could look inside themselves, they would have also noticed an entire cascade of events taking place; changes lowering their blood pressure, increasing oxygen to the brain, reducing dangerous inflammation, and jacking their immune system to new heights. All these benefits were occurring because they were giving and receiving love.

Love is not something added to the human existence to help fight disease. Love was here long before. Love is the governing power behind all creation. It drives the unseen machinery of the universe and makes possible the laws holding it in place. How do we know this? Let me share an amazing text found in God's Holy Word. Think of the implications for your life as you read it. "Whoever does not love does not know God, because God is love" (1 John 4:8).

This Bible writer does not say God loves, or God needs to be loved. He simply states God *is* love. Our heavenly "Team" (God the Father, God the Son, and God the Holy Spirit) functions from a foundation of love. Everything They say, everything They do, and every plan They make springs from a well of pure, undefiled love. God cannot operate any other way. Keep this fact in mind the next time you sit down to read your Bible. It will transform your understanding of God's Word and His place in your life.

So, if love governs the universe, and love was the driving force behind the creation of this world, should it surprise us that love is a healing element in our lives? We were built for love. We are also maintained by love. And it will be love that sustains us for eternity.

Further proof of this is demonstrated when love is lost. It is common knowledge among cardiologists that when a loved one dies suddenly, a perfectly healthy spouse can experience surges in epinephrine, a condition that can cause a heart attack. It's called the "broken heart syndrome." I have seen this condition three times in the past five years. The arteries are without blockages and the blood is flowing freely. Then the loss causes an extreme stress on the body. The resultant chemical changes precipitate a heart attack. Also, when a spouse passes, the remaining partner is much more likely to develop health problems even if he or she was previously healthy. There is a change of chemistry when love is removed. Some are able to recover from the loss and rebuild their lives. Some cannot, and they actually die of a broken heart.

Which brings us back to my two dogs. When human love is not readily available, pets can help improve a person's health as well. Those who allow an animal or two into their lives experience less heart attacks, infections, and need fewer medications. It takes love to recover from the loss of love. Nothing else is as powerful and long lasting.

The Opposite of Love

Love changes body chemistry for the good. Conversely, selfishness—the very opposite of love—changes body chemistry for the worse. Living a life centered on your own needs, your own desires, and your own specifications introduces dangerous chemical changes. Am I saying the lack of love in this world is a determining factor in our present health crises? Am I saying selfishness is just as destructive to the human body as eating low-fiber, high-fat, highly processed foods, living a sedentary lifestyle, and filling our minds with the filth the media makes so readily available? Yes, that is *exactly* what I am saying. Selfishness is definitely present in this world at many levels and is causing many of the stressors leading to disease and the need for acute-care modern medicine.

When Lucifer brought selfishness into God's perfect universe of love (remember, true love allows choices to be made), our present health-care dilemma began. Selfishness was not a law governing the universe. It was, in reality, an "anti-law." It generated stress, and this stress set in motion all the negative chemical reactions with which we battle to this day. We were created to be with God; to live our lives encircled, supported, and sustained by His love. But Adam and Eve chose to turn their backs on God. They switched paths, and began heading down the road leading to eternal death. The bottom line? They chose to live separated from God, separated from the source of true love, and separated from the healing power driving the universe. Human genetics became altered, body chemistry changed dramatically, chronic diseases developed, and death became everyone's ultimate destination. That is the end result when one lives apart from God. That is what happens when one lives outside of the powerful forces of life-sustaining love.

But it was the very force—the force of love—that handed a compass to a lost humanity. "For God so loved the world that he gave his one and only Son, that whoever believes in him shall not perish but have eternal life" (John 3:16). God gave us the ultimate expression of love when He gave His Son.

"This is how God showed his love among us: He sent his one and only Son into the world that we might live through him." This is the antidote. "This is love: not that we loved God, but that he loved us and sent his Son as an atoning sacrifice for our sins. . . . Since God so loved us, we also ought to love one another" (1 John 4:9-11).

Love is the solution to our global health-care dilemma. Love opens the door for us to rediscover the heart of health and find healing for our minds, bodies, and spirits. Love is the ultimate treatment. It is the final step to a full, long-lasting recovery.

But the evil one wants us to be deceived into thinking we cannot find love on this earth; we cannot find happiness in a growing relationship with God. He is saying to us, "God does not love you! You must find other means to be healed. You must depend solely on certain sets of medications, specific doctrines, good deeds, the proper diet, giving your money to the poor, and living your life as others define it." The deception first spoken in Eden continues to echo in our minds and hearts today: "You will not surely die." And we're taking the bait.

However, now you know better. Now you have discovered the heart of health and are ready to introduce this amazingly powerful "medicine" into your life. When you do, you will experience—perhaps for the first time ever—the healing properties God placed within this divine law.

So, get ready to continue your journey to optimum health. This final step will bring you a degree of healing you never dreamed possible!

Chapter 18

Ultimate Healing

One day a young woman walked into a fabric shop and hurried to the counter. "Excuse me, sir," she said to the owner. "I'm looking for some noisy, rustling, white material."

The proprietor thought for a moment, then guided his customer across the room to where several bundles of cloth lay on a shelf. "How about these?" he asked.

Wordlessly, the woman picked up the first bolt, unfolded a few feet of the fabric, and shook it vigorously while listening carefully. She did the same for the next bolt, and the next. Finally, she smiled. "This one," she announced. "This cloth is perfect."

As the owner was measuring out the length of fabric his customer had requested, curiosity got the best of him. "If I may be so bold," he said, "may I ask why you want *noisy* cloth?"

The woman smiled shyly. "You see, sir, I'm making my wedding gown, and my fiancé is blind. When I walk down the aisle, I want him to know when I've arrived at the altar, so he won't be embarrassed."

What love! What tender regard! And what a perfect description of how God sometimes operates in our lives. There are moments when He gets downright noisy in His attempts to reveal His love for us. Just ask the children of Israel staring up at Mount Sinai. Just ask the guards on Calvary staring up at a dying Christ amid ground-shaking peals of thunder. Just ask Saul on the road to Damascus staring up into a vortex of wind and light as God speaks to him. Yes, sometimes love must shout!

But there are other times when God's love is revealed to us in less dramatic ways—when we find Him in the "still, small voice" that Elijah heard while hiding in a cave. God never stops trying. Whether His voice is noisy or still, He's always speaking to those who are willing to listen to His words of affection and guidance. I pray that you're listening now.

Different Futures

We've identified two paths—two very different ways of living with two very different futures. One path is tied directly into Creation and the laws God set in place during that incredible week. The other path follows the father of all deception—the devil—as he has been luring men and women away from a loving relationship with their heavenly Father. One path is all about health, good chemistry, and life. The other is all about sickness, bad chemistry, and death.

Here's the question we need to ask ourselves: "How do I really know which path I'm on?"

The answer has to do with symptoms. As a cardiologist, I am very interested in the whole concept of symptoms because they reveal so much about the underlying disease from which my patients may be suffering. If I have a clear understanding of their symptoms, I can do a pretty good job of forming a diagnosis.

Chest pains? Possibly restricted blood flow to the heart. Dizziness and fainting? Might be not enough oxygen reaching the brain. Shortness of breath? Numbness in the arm? Confusion? Slurred speech? All are clues indicating something serious and unseen is taking place inside the body.

The two paths generate symptoms as well. On God's path—when we are living in harmony with His *spiritual* laws, laws governing the universe—we are more hopeful, confident, and accepting of others' faults. We find it easier to forgive, forget, and move on.

On Satan's path, the spiritual picture is quite different. It's here where our hearts and bodies fill with despair, anger, resentment, and unrelenting guilt. On this pathway, we live in fear of the very God who longs to save us from our sinful selves.

There's a *physical* component to this journey as well. It is only on God's path that we find true healing. Optimum health is not dependent on some prescription drug or miracle cure. It is not available over the counter or online. Optimum health is what happens when we live in harmony with God's health laws.

What are the physical symptoms of traveling along the path of deception—of turning our backs on what God intended when He created us? They can include lifestyle-related conditions such as diabetes, heart disease, obesity, cancers, and shortened life spans. Even God-loving people who enjoy a rich and rewarding relationship with their Creator can suffer greatly from these lifestyle diseases and end up in early graves if they refuse to follow God's Health Plan. They find themselves depending on modern medicine or the incredible pressure of appetite to form the foundation of their lives. When it comes to their physical health, they walk the wrong path and pay dearly for their choices. I see it all the time.

Conversely, there are those who come into my office who follow Eden's ideal to the letter, yet suffer from many of the same illnesses as their spiritual brothers and sisters do. Why? Because they refuse to allow love, the spirit of God, to rule in their lives. They eat the right foods, yet hate their neighbor. They exercise daily, yet cheat on their taxes. They breathe in plenty of fresh air and drink ample amounts of pure water, yet fill their minds with the senseless and violent content the modern media makes so readily available.

The point I am trying to make is this: our spiritual and physical lives cannot operate independently of each other. We cannot walk on both God's and Satan's path at the same time and expect good results. The interconnection between the mind and the body is so overpowering, that trying to serve both masters brings only disaster.

This describes my patient David. He loved his family and attended church regularly, yet he strolled merrily along the path of deception when it came to his physical health. Obeying all of the Ten Commandments won't do a thing to save you if your eating habits are clogging up your arteries. You can shut yourself up in a monastery and pray 24 hours a day, but you can die young of obesity-related diseases because you didn't get any exercise. You simply cannot live your life with one foot on God's path and the other foot on Satan's path and expect to enjoy optimum health. It's not going to happen. You have to place both feet firmly on God's path if you hope to live a healthy life. There is no other way.

So, where does the heart of health come in? What part does love play in this incredible drama? The answer is simple . . . and beautiful. The heart of health is what motivates—and provides the power for—us to change paths. It's where we discover love for the God who made us and find the strength to stop believing deceptive lies about Him. It's where we learn to love those we serve, even if some are unkind and ungenerous toward us. Most important, it's where we learn to love ourselves as children of God. Someone who is filled with this type of love would never knowingly do anything to harm others . . . or self—including breaking God's health laws.

We are often taught to concentrate on others more than ourselves. There is certainly wisdom in this concept. But there is a danger, too. To enjoy optimum health, we've got to learn to love ourselves. We've got to believe God when He tells us, through the apostle Paul: "Do you not know that your body is a temple of the Holy Spirit, who is in you, whom you have received from God? You are not your own; you were bought at a price. Therefore honor God with your body" (1 Corinthians 6:19, 20).

Knowing this, what are you putting into your mind and body temple? Does your life and your body honor God? Do you have both feet planted firmly on the right path or do you need to make some changes in your life? Are you on your way to experiencing ultimate healing?

A Matter of Worship

Probably the most profound question we need to ask ourselves when it comes to experiencing longed-for ultimate healing is "Whom do we worship?"

Worship takes many forms—all of which affect our chemistry. Our worship may include a weekly church service. It might be out in nature, taking a walk, watching a sunset, listening to the ocean, smelling the fresh air, or seeing a smile. Worship might be helping a friend, offering a thankful prayer, singing a song, or writing a letter.

This may surprise you, but we actually become like that which we worship—that is how profound worship is to our minds and bodies. If we spend time communing with God, we become more like God—seeing life through His eyes, responding to situations as He'd respond—all of which bring healing forces into our body. But, if we bow at Satan's altar, we worship other "things," we become selfish, angry, fearful—emotions that damage the body and can undo many of the good things we do for it.

Here is the most exciting part. As we worship God, we begin to better understand the world and our place in it based on truth, not lies. We learn to avoid deception. We find we have the power to make the changes those truths demand—the very truths I have tried to introduce to you in this book. We discover the proper place for modern medicine and for alternate ways of healing. We actually enjoy the process of exploring new avenues for bringing sound nutrition and intelligent exercise into our lives. We begin to change outwardly . . . and inwardly. Our chemistry adjusts to the new way of living and we find we feel better, sleep better, and experience a closer walk with God.

Then something absolutely miraculous happens. When we put the interests of others above our own, we become healers—bringing healing hope to the minds and bodies of those around us. They, in turn, become healers within their circle of influence—the home, the church, the community. We all become "healing missionaries," changing the chemistry of countless people—everyone from the teenager behind the counter at the grocery store to the struggling neighbor who lives down the street. The love we share acts like a powerful medicine, easing heartaches and pain, motivating people to return to the source of ultimate healing. There is no drug, no medical procedure, no treatment that can accomplish this degree of restoration. The heart of health acts like an energizing force in countless lives, transforming people in ways they never thought possible.

But don't expect your healing ministry to be easy or universally accepted. The heart of health must be strong.

What Is Right

I always enjoy my visits with Roland. A few years ago, he underwent a successful surgery on his stenotic mitral valve. Since his surgery, he has continued to do well, is on a blood thinner to help lower the risk of stroke, and takes another medication to help control the speed of his atrial fibrillation—modern medicine at its best.

Over the years Roland has made the slow adjustment to retirement. For a man who was in ministry in every corner of the world, being away from the front lines of evangelism has been quite a challenge.

Recently, he came in for a physical and checked out just fine. During our conversation, I mentioned this book and how I felt the Spirit of God leading me to write about what some are thinking but few dare say. I described the possible backlash I would experience because I was stepping on a lot of toes within my own profession. The powers that be would probably not be enthralled by a book that pointed to the Great Physician as the true source of all healing, and I shared my concern that my book might fail to reach those who needed it the most.

Roland thought for a moment, then told me this story.

He was in a very important leadership position when his grandson was born. However, he found himself wanting to spend as much time as possible with the little boy. Sometimes, because he was taking time to be part of his grandson's life, he would arrive a little late for meetings at work.

One day Roland walked into the busy day-care center to pick up his grandson. The room was full of people and noise. The child, even though he was across the room, sensed the man's presence and, despite the chaos, moved toward his grandfather. Their eyes locked, and the little one cried out the word "Papa" with great love. This was the first time the little boy had ever spoken.

As Roland told me the story, I could see tears of joy in his eyes. Then he looked at me and said, "Jim, you have to do what is right even if no one else in the world understands but you and God. The long-term rewards are always worth it when you put love for others first. People may not understand you, but in the end, following the Spirit's leading is the ultimate gratification."

I needed to hear that.

When we love, when we make someone laugh, when we help someone along life's way, we are giving that person a great prescription. We are literally changing their chemistry; we're flooding their system with endorphins as we lower their levels of adrenaline and other harmful elements. We are helping to heal them. We are sharing the heart of love.

Roland related to me how he had worked with great healers all over the world. These were medical missionaries who gladly served, contented to grow in the places God had planted them. I decided then and there I want to incorporate Roland's vision of service into, not only my cardiology practice, but also my life. I want to be content in whatever place I'm called to serve. I want to help heal a diseased world. And more than that, someday I want to see my heavenly "Papa" and run into His arms, because I know He took the time and made the necessary sacrifices to teach me how to love.

The Long Journey

I have many people come to my office to just ask questions because they have concerns. It might be worries about a leaky valve, a question about a medication, or the fear about an "unusual feeling" they're experiencing in their chest. When their concerns are heard, when they learn the truth—no matter how simple or complex it may be—they feel reassured. This reassurance makes them feel better as the doubt that was creating a negative chemical environment deep inside them is replaced by the peace of knowing the truth.

Our Great Physician is waiting to reassure us. He wants to demonstrate His love and let us know He is constantly available to help keep us on the right path—on His path. Most of all, He wants us to come to know true love, and this can only occur as we maintain a daily relationship with Him. This interaction with our Creator helps our chemistry and allows our doubts and fears to vanish. Peace floods our hearts and health floods our bodies.

This amazing relationship was originally formed in the Garden of Eden as God revealed His love for Adam and Eve. The animals, the plants, the work needing to be done, God's health laws; all were manifestations of this loving relationship. There were no doubts, no bad chemistry, no need for healing, no stress. Love ruled the day.

But those two beings opened the door for deception to enter the world, and everything changed. They believed the lies, and immediately selfishness and doubts entered their hearts. The perfect world began its long journey toward oblivion.

As time moved on, deceptions took root in our culture. Perceptions of God changed. The evil one constantly fed the world a diet of doubts and misconceptions—lies that have been passed down through the generations. In an attempt to reestablish His lost relationship with us, God provided laws to remind us what love looked like. He called forth spokespeople to keep us on track. But few listened.

Finally, He sent us His Son to personally reconnect us with the only true source of ultimate healing. Even though we hung Him on the cross, the message remains.

Today, we are in the midst of Satan's final deception—a false sense of security generated by our almost total dependence on modern medicine, high-tech science, and a belief that the answers we seek can be found in our own intelligence.

But God wants us to know the truth. He walks through the garden of our lives calling our names, inviting us to join Him on the path leading to ultimate healing.

Right now, at this moment, wherever you are, answer the call. Allow the Holy Spirit to take control, not only of your thoughts, but of how you care for your body. Enter into a fresh, new, exciting, healing relationship with your heavenly Father. "Here I am!" God says in Revelation 3:20. "I stand at the door and knock. If anyone hears my voice and opens the door, I will go in and eat with him, and he with me."

The Creator is waiting and wanting to lead you back to the original plan He established at Creation. He is waiting to help you break away from deceptions and return to a worship of the one true God. He is waiting to walk with you on your journey to optimum health.

There is hope for the sickest person. There is hope for those who suffer with chronic pain. There is hope for incurable disease. There is hope for those who have chosen through the years to ignore how they were designed to live. This hope is in a relationship with our Creator who will bring us back to truths, revealing deception at every level of life. This relationship will bring us back to the heart of health—love, the governing force in the universe. No matter where you are on this journey, that relationship will be there with you keeping you on the right path.

Come back to love. Choose now to embrace and enjoy the eternal benefits found only at the heart of health.

Symptoms

M any people have or will have problems with their hearts. Therefore, a basic explanation of what that looks and feels like will enhance the understanding of the medical jargon they'll hear as they fight to regain health.

When a part of a system is not functioning correctly, sooner or later problems develop. A car with a hole in its gas tank may run for a while, but eventually it must stop. A vacuum cleaner will not work without a belt. A dishwasher will have problems cleaning dishes without soap. Similarly, if the cardiovascular system is not working correctly, sooner or later problems will develop.

Mr. Gregory, 52, was, and still is, an active man. But for the past six months, he has felt something different inside. Lately, those feelings have been coming on more frequently.

In the evening he walks his dog. There's a small hill in the middle of their route through the neighborhood. Every time Mr. Gregory walks up the hill, he feels a heavy sensation in his chest. He also experiences shortness of breath. Six months ago he could make it up the hill without any problem at all, but now he stops five or six times before reaching the top.

Mr. Gregory is experiencing mild to moderate symptoms. *Symptoms* are feelings that are not normal for an individual, or a change in an individual's condition. Mr. Gregory eventually got help, but he took a chance by waiting.

Wayne O'Neal, a corporate lawyer, was at work early one morning. While preparing for a conference, he experienced severe chest pain. After collapsing, he was rushed to the Emergency Department of a local hospital. Mr. O'Neal was experiencing *severe* symptoms.

Unfortunately, many of us wait too long to find help when something "isn't right." The cardiovascular system is wonderfully made, but nothing is perfect. The system can break down under certain circumstances. How do we know when there's a problem? Hopefully, a *symptom* will be our first clue. Mr. O'Neal had no choice but to get help.

Mr. Scott, 65, had just retired and was planning a vacation to the Pacific Northwest. He was fairly active and did some farming; however, he had not felt well for two months. He was tired, couldn't catch his breath, and noticed his legs swelling.

His family tried to get him to see the doctor, but he had other "more important" things to do.

One day, while in the fields, he collapsed. Tragically, when he arrived in the Emergency Department, his heart had stopped. The medical team could not help him.

My point is this: We must pay close attention to our bodies. When something is not right, we need to consider this as a warning sign and seek help. Also, if you know others who are having problems, encourage them to seek help sooner rather than later. It's easier to deal with a small problem than a catastrophe.

Each individual is unique; everyone feels differently when the cardiovascular system is not working well. Not every person with heart disease will have a symptom. People without obvious symptoms are the most difficult to help and evaluate. Actually, the people without symptoms are more likely to notice that they do not feel "normal." This may be their symptom.

Let's review the more common symptoms that occur when the cardiovascular system malfunctions.

Chest Pain

Chest pain is a very common symptom of cardiovascular disease. It can come from many different sources, including the heart. One might not feel "classic" pain. But a discomfort or "funny feeling" in the chest, arms, jaw, neck, teeth, and even the back could be related to the heart. The discomfort might be squeezing or pressing in nature. In my years as a cardiologist, I have heard pain described in many different ways, but always I hear, "Something isn't right."

Angina is used to describe a condition of discomfort caused by decreased blood flow to the heart. These abnormal feelings may mean the heart is not getting enough blood.

I once saw a gentleman with angina in the back. Sometimes discomfort in the stomach indicates angina. Often, patients think they have indigestion, when in reality this is pain related to the heart. Discomfort, brought on consistently by exertion, strong emotions, or even after a big meal, is a particular concern.

Sometimes pain or discomfort lasts for long periods of time. In this case, an individual could be experiencing a heart attack. A heart attack results when the blood flow supplying nourishment to the heart is cut off completely. Some say a heart attack feels like an elephant is sitting on the chest. However, a heart attack can feel many different ways. The pain or discomfort might start in the front of the chest and move to the arm, neck, jaw, stomach, or back. There might be other feelings, including shortness of breath, weakness, dizziness, sickness of the stomach, sweating, feeling an abnormal heartbeat and/or clammy skin.

However, all prolonged chest pain is not necessarily a heart attack or angina. In fact, acid in the stomach, sprained chest muscles, problems with the lungs, esophagus, and other internal conditions can cause pain or discomfort in the upper body as well.

Nevertheless, I want you to think that something might not be right with the heart when these symptoms appear. If you experience these symptoms, call 911 and get help right away. Never drive yourself to the hospital; this would put you, and others, at great risk.

I want to reemphasize that chest pain can present itself in a variety of ways. I often hear excuses like . . .

- It's just heartburn.
- I'm too young to have a heart problem.
- The pain is not too bad—I'll just wait to see if it goes away.
- I don't think this is my heart.
- I'm too busy to get help.
- I don't want to be a bother to my family.
- It's the middle of the night—I'll wait till morning.
- No one in my family has had heart problems.

Don't make excuses. The sooner you get help, the better. It is *not* embarrassing to ask for help. It may save your life.

Heart Racing

A racing heart might represent a problem. Sometimes you might feel a fluttering, a skipping, a heavy pounding, or a jumpy feeling. Others may call these symptoms *palpitations*.

Dizziness, Light-headedness, Passing Out

Though many conditions can cause these feelings, they can be associated with serious heart conditions. In particular, the electrical system may not be working well. It's imperative that the possible causes of these abnormal feelings be evaluated.

Collapse

This is a very serious problem that warrants immediate medical attention and could be life-threatening.

Shortness of Breath

Dyspnea is the medical term for shortness of breath. This could represent a cardiovascular malfunction. Sometimes an individual unknowingly restricts activities because he/she cannot get a good breath. Typically, it is difficult to sort out why an individual is short of breath, because many different conditions can cause this feeling. For example, physical exertion in a nonactive person can cause dyspnea. But a prolonged period of dyspnea could be a sign of a larger problem.

Swelling

The medical term for this symptom is *edema*. Fluid may collect in the legs, hands or abdomen. At times, fluid can collect in the lungs, which could cause shortness of breath.

Unusual Fatigue

Feeling tired much of the time may represent a medical problem and should be evaluated by a doctor.

Coughing

Prolonged coughing episodes or unexplainable coughing associated with lying down need to be evaluated. An adverse heart condition could be the cause.

Unable to Breathe Comfortably When Lying Flat

The medical term for this condition is *orthopnea*. This could be related to the heart.

Skin Discoloration

If the skin has a bluish color, this could be a sign of inadequate blood flow that might indicate a heart malfunction.

Headache

This is a common symptom I hear about daily. A headache could be related to cardiovascular disease; the blood pressure might be elevated.

Other Symptoms

I want to emphasize that some groups of people—for example, diabetics and the elderly—may experience mild or unusual symptoms, making a heart problem more difficult to detect. Also, females do not often have the typical symptoms of "chest pain."

If you're experiencing the symptoms mentioned here, I hope you've already been evaluated by a doctor. The sooner a problem is analyzed, the better.

The following chart gives common symptoms related to the heart, the possible abnormality causing the symptom, and the general medical term describing the cardiac abnormality.

SYMPTOM	POSSIBLE CARDIOVASCULAR SYSTEM ABNORMALITY (1)	GENERAL MEDICAL TERM
Chest pain (2)	Complete blockage of a coronary artery leading to the heart	Myocardial infarction (heart attack)
	Partial blockage	Angina
	Opening and closing of a coronary artery	Coronary spasm
	Inflammation of the outside lining of the heart	Pericarditis
	Abnormality of a heart valve	Mitral valve prolapse or aortic stenosis
	Tear in the large artery (aorta) leaving the heart	Dissection
	Abnormal fast beating of the heart; an electrical system abnormality	Tachyarrhythmia (3)

SYMPTOM	POSSIBLE CARDIOVASCULAR SYSTEM ABNORMALITY (1)	GENERAL MEDICAL TERM
Shortness of breath (dyspnea)	Complete blockage of a coronary artery	Myocardial infarction
	Partial blockage of a coronary artery	Angina
	Abnormality in the heart valves	Valvular heart disease Mitral regurgitation Mitral stenosis Aortic regurgitation Aortic stenosis
	Heart beating too slow or too fast	Bradyarrhythmia or Tachyarrhythmia (3)
	Weak heart muscle	Cardiomyopathy

SYMPTOM	POSSIBLE CARDIOVASCULAR SYSTEM ABNORMALITY (1)	GENERAL MEDICAL TERM
Dizziness, Loss of consciousness, or passing out	Heart going too slow or too fast	Bradyarrhythmia or Tachyarrhythmia
	Complete blockage or partial blockage of a coronary artery	Myocardial infarction or angina
	Heart valve not opening	Aortic stenosis
	Artery blockage in neck vessel (brain does not get enough blood with oxygen)	Cerebral vascular accident or stroke (4)
Swelling (edema)	Heart muscle weak (5)	Cardiomyopathy
Heart racing, or palpitations	Abnormality in electrical system	Tachyarrhythmia (3)
Unusual fatigue (6)	Weak heart	Cardiomyopathy
	Abnormal electrical system (heart going too fast or too slow)	Tachyarrhythmia or Bradyarrythmia (3)

SYMPTOM	POSSIBLE CARDIOVASCULAR SYSTEM ABNORMALITY (1)	GENERAL MEDICAL TERM
Coughing (7)	Fluid building up in lungs	Pulmonary edema
Unable to breathe comfortably when lying down (orthopnea)	Fluid building up in lungs (8)	Pulmonary edema
Headache (9)	High pressure in the arteries	Hypertension (10)
Skin Discoloration (11)	Insufficient blood with oxygen in body	

1. The abnormalities listed have been limited to the more common malfunctions of the cardiovascular system. The origin of the abnormality has not been specified.
2. There are many causes of chest pain that are unrelated to the cardiovascular system, but it is beyond the scope of this book to list them all.
3. There are many different types of fast heart rates (*tachyarrhythmias*) and slow heart rates (*bradyarrhythmias*).
4. More discussion in a later chapter.
5. There are numerous reasons that a heart muscle can be weak. For more information, see the appendix references.

6. There are many other causes of fatigue unrelated to the cardiovascular system.
7. There are many other noncardiac causes of a cough, from a simple cold to sinus drainage.
8. There could also be other causes.
9. Headache has many other noncardiovascular causes.
10. Hypertension typically has no symptoms.
11. There are numerous causes of skin discoloration, including the heart is not pumping blood to the body, or the connections in the cardiovascular system are wrong. This is usually an abnormality occurring at birth (*congenital*) and is often detected at an early age.

When a symptom is discovered, you may need an evaluation, which may include diagnostic testing. There are many ways to evaluate symptoms. Unfortunately, sometimes this is not an easy task. It's important to see a doctor or other health-care provider who can help.

Diagnostic Testing

Tom Gentry, 46, is a hardworking mechanic. Most say he's the best in town. He'd seen a physician about 10 months before coming to my office. Tom wasn't a talkative person, but I could tell he would not be seeing me unless something was wrong.

During the course of our conversation, he told me a previous doctor had wanted to "put me through the mill." He decided to risk dying rather than "be tortured by tests." I spent a long time convincing him that none of our testing was torture. Some tests might be a little uncomfortable, but knowing the cause of his symptoms, in my opinion, would be worth the risk of the testing. After that, Tom said, "Couldn't I just have a pill to make me all better?"

I wish it were that simple. I explained to him that testing would help me know the cause of the problem. Once we identified the cause, we could give the right treatment. This might include medications, surgery, or factors in his lifestyle that needed changing.

To make a long story short, Tom went through several tests. I was careful to explain why each was performed and what to expect during the routines. I explained the risks. This knowledge seemed to help my patient tremendously. Understanding the tests decreased some of his fears and gave him confidence and a feeling of being in control. Eventually, Tom underwent heart surgery. This, along with some important lifestyle changes, returned my patient to a normal and productive life.

There are many methods by which your health-care provider may evaluate your symptoms for heart disease. Here are a few of the most common procedures used in diagnostic testing. It all begins with words.

Evaluation Process

In the evaluation process, your health-care provider will listen to and talk with you first. Hopefully you can describe, in detail, what makes you feel "not right." More questions might follow. This discussion can provide more information than the most advanced tests. The provider will ask questions regarding past medical problems and treatments. Having an up-to-date health record is important in helping both you and the provider to understand the entire picture. If you're seeing a new provider, please bring your old records. It will expedite your care.

Physical Examination

When the interview phase is completed, the provider is thinking, *What could be causing this feeling?* The next step will be a physical examination. The provider is trying to obtain more information. I consider the interview and the exam the most important parts in making a correct *diagnosis* (the medical term explaining the symptoms). The physical exam will include the provider observing you and your body, and taking your vital signs. Measuring the vital signs consists of feeling or listening to how fast your heart is going per minute, counting how many times you breathe in a minute, measuring the body temperature and blood pressure. The provider obtains your blood pressure by listening for sounds in your blood vessels while using a device to squeeze your upper arm. This will measure the pressure in the cardiovascular system. This test is slightly uncomfortable because a device squeezes the arm, but it is certainly not unbearable.

Next, your body will be examined and listened to. Skilled examiners are efficient, so this does not take too long, and there are really no risks or discomforts. The physical exam gives even more clues in finding the cause of your symptoms. Sometimes a cause will be found and no further tests will be needed.

Further Tests

After talking to you and examining your body, the health-care provider will decide if further tests are needed; and if so, what specific tests would be most beneficial.

Following is an explanation of the most common tests used to evaluate the cardiovascular system.

Electrocardiogram (EKG or ECG)

This is a recording of the heart's electrical impulses. The test gives much information, including the rhythm of the heart, evidence of a heart attack, and thickening of the heart muscle. It could also aid in determining whether the heart is getting enough blood.

The test lasts about five minutes and is performed by placing small patches at specific locations on the chest, arms, and legs. These small patches are called electrodes. Usually the individual is lying down during the test. The data is recorded on special paper.

If a chest is hairy, some of the hair may need to be shaved so that the electrode has better contact with the skin. This test has no significant risks or dangers. Rarely, there might be a slight skin reaction when the body is shaved before the leads are placed.

Blood Work

There are times when blood is drawn, usually from the arm, and sent to the lab for analysis. Blood analysis gives information about the function of many of the internal organs. Troponin and Creatinine Phosphokinase (CPK) are common blood tests that help determine if a heart muscle is dying or not getting enough nourishment.

Usually, the cholesterol level is measured. When this is done, the individual should be without food for 12 hours prior to the time blood is drawn. *Atrial natriuretic peptide* is another blood test used to evaluate if the heart is working efficiently.

To draw blood, usually a tourniquet is placed on the arm above a vein. A needle is inserted into the vein and the blood is removed. The test time is less than a minute if a vein is easily found. Before the needle is placed, the entire area is cleaned to help prevent infection. There is a very small chance of bleeding, and some pain occurs (varies from person to person) when the needle breaks the skin.

When a small sterile plastic device is placed into a vein, this is called an IV (intravenous). This device is usually inserted in the arm or wrist. Tubing is attached that allows fluid and medication to be given directly into the bloodstream for immediate action.

THE HEART OF HEALTH: AVOIDING DECEPTION

Echocardiography

In an echocardiogram, sound waves bounce off the various structures of the heart and a picture is constructed. The moving picture gives a wealth of information that includes the structure and strength of your heart, as well as the blood flow within the heart. The test might reveal if there has been a previous heart attack. The heart valves are also evaluated.

First, two or three electrodes are placed on the chest to monitor the heart rhythm. A small device called a *transducer* is placed at different locations on the chest wall. Sound waves are sent from this device, thus creating the picture. The patient usually lies on his or her left side on a special bed that has an area cut out so the transducer can be easily manipulated. Don't worry, the patient is covered for privacy.

The sonographer (person who obtains the pictures) will place the transducer, along with some gel, on the chest wall. The gel aids in obtaining the best pictures. The sonographer will change the position of the transducer many times during the test to look at the heart from a variety of angles. The images are permanently recorded on videotape or disc.

Sometimes the pushing feels uncomfortable. Some describe a tickling feeling. There's no preparation needed and there are no significant risks to this test.

Holter Monitor

This test records every beat of the heart for 24 to 48 hours and helps to determine whether the heart's electrical system is malfunctioning. For example, the monitor will detect whether the heart is going too fast or too slow, skipping a beat, or even stopping. You will be asked to write in a diary the specific times you feel differently and the way you're feeling. The health-care provider can correlate symptoms with the heart's electrical system.

The individual wears a small monitoring device, usually placed on a belt around the waist. The device records the action of the heart and is attached to electrodes placed in a similar manner as in an EKG.

No specific preparation is needed. The risks are minimal to none.

Event Monitor

There are times when an individual has only occasional symptoms. The *event monitor* records the heart rhythm up to a month at a time. It's a device similar to the Holter monitor in terms of placement. When a symptom occurs, the patient activates the device and the heart rhythm is recorded for a short period. The information is usually sent immediately to the health-care provider. A diary is also given to the patient.

I once had a patient with very infrequent symptoms. I could not "catch" the symptoms on a Holter or event monitor. Today, there are small devices that can be implanted below the skin in the chest wall to record every single heartbeat for as long as a year. For my patient, I recommended using this device, and sure enough, in a few months he felt symptoms. We discovered the type of electrical malfunction he suffered, which was one that could be easily treated. These devices are rarely used, but I did want to mention their availability.

Exercise Stress Test

In this test, stress is placed on the heart usually by exercising, or sometimes by pedaling a bicycle. The provider monitors changes in the cardiovascular system by using a continuous EKG, checking the blood pressure frequently, and evaluating symptoms and exercise ability during the stress.

An exercise stress test gives information on whether there is adequate blood flow to the heart during conditions when the heart works harder. The level of cardiovascular fitness can also be estimated.

If the individual can walk, an exercise stress is used. The patient walks on a treadmill that increases in speed and incline over a period of time. A stationary bicycle can also be used in some situations. Exercise increases the heart rate. The provider monitors the EKG and asks frequently whether symptoms are developing. Blood pressure is measured often.

The stress test requires an individual to be without food before the test, to wear comfortable walking clothes and shoes, and to be able to walk or pedal at increasing speeds. The risks are small. The main risk is developing symptoms while walking. I tell my patients, "I would rather have you develop a symptom with me watching where I could do something, rather than develop symptoms at home." A skin irritation could also occur, owing to the electrode placement.

Some patients are unable to walk adequately on a treadmill. In this case, there are other types of nonexercise stress tests. These will be discussed shortly.

Stress Echocardiogram

In addition to the information obtained from a regular stress test, a stress echocardiogram gives pictures of the heart before and after exercise. The provider looks to see if the heart muscle performs differently after exercise. This added information gives an additional tool to detect problems.

The test begins with an echocardiogram, as previously described. The patient then walks on a treadmill. After the walk, while the heart is still beating fast, another set of pictures of the heart is obtained. These images, in addition to the information gained during the regular stress test, are reviewed to detect abnormalities. The risks and preparation for the test are as described for the stress test and echocardiogram.

Nuclear Medicine Stress Test

A nuclear medicine stress test adds a different element to the normal stress test and enhances diagnostic abilities. As with the other stress tests, the blood flow to the heart muscle is evaluated.

In addition to the stress test, a radioactive material (Thallium or Cardiolite) is injected into a vein. The radioactive tracer travels throughout the heart and helps to evaluate blood flow.

The test is usually done in two stages. First, images are made of blood flow to the heart. For this, the patient lies flat and an X-ray machine takes pictures at different angles.

Next, the patient exercises. Again, a radioactive tracer is injected. More images are obtained after the exercise. The provider then compares blood flows before the exercise to the flow after the exercise. The comparison assists in detection of possible problems.

In preparation, the provider will ask the patient not to have food for at least six hours before the test. The patient must also abstain from caffeine for 48 hours before the test. This is hard for some because caffeine is in many items that people eat and drink. The provider may ask the patient to hold certain medications, especially if these medications would affect the speed of the heart or the patient's ability to exercise. Diabetics will receive special instructions regarding their blood sugar medications. As with the regular stress test, casual clothes are recommended, along with shoes appropriate for walking. The entire test lasts about three hours.

The risks are similar to those of the regular stress test, but with the added minimal risk of starting an IV and the rare chance of an adverse reaction to the radioactive material. There is also a very small risk of exposure to radiation. The actual radiation received is less than you would receive from having a regular chest X-ray.

Gated Scanning

Sometimes a nuclear stress test includes gated scanning. This test helps determine the overall strength, or pumping ability, of the heart. This scan is frequently used to evaluate whether medications—especially medications used to fight cancer—are weakening the heart muscle.

The test is performed by placing a radioactive tracer in the blood via an IV that circulates to the heart. The pumping ability is then determined by taking pictures of the heart with a nuclear camera. The risks and preparation are similar to those for the nuclear stress test.

Nonexercise Stress Tests

When an individual is unable to walk on a treadmill, another type of stress to the heart might be needed. These tests involve use of medications (dobutamine) that speed up the heart, or medications (adenosine or Persantine, just to name two) that cause the coronary arteries to become bigger. These agents are injected into a vein via an IV. The examination evaluates blood flow to the heart before and after the stress that these agents provide. The EKG, blood pressure, and symptoms are monitored continually during the testing.

Before the medication is injected into a vein, X-ray pictures are made of the heart—the same as for a regular nuclear examination. The prone patient is under constant monitoring while the medication is injected. Another set of X-ray pictures of the heart is taken 15 to 30 minutes later. Both sets of pictures are compared to evaluate if the heart is getting sufficient blood. The images are stored on computer discs.

The risks are small and include those of the regular nuclear test. Also, there is the risk of an adverse reaction to the medication given to stress the heart. Again, the risks are small compared to the benefit of a diagnosis. The preparation is usually the same as for the nuclear test. Your provider will guide you as to which medications to take or avoid before the test.

Transesophageal Echocardiogram (TEE)

In this examination, a small device called a *probe* is passed into the swallowing tube, or esophagus. The *esophagus* is a tube located behind your heart that takes food from your mouth to your stomach. From the vantage point of the esophagus, a device can obtain clear pictures of the heart. The information obtained is similar to that offered by an echocardiogram. The TEE is used when clear pictures of the heart cannot be obtained from the transthoracic (chest) views.

Sometimes this test is used when a patient has suffered injury to the chest wall or has an extremely large chest. This test can also give specific information on valvular structure and function because it can also visualize parts of the heart that a regular echocardiogram cannot evaluate well.

Why not perform this test on everyone if the pictures are so clear? The test is more uncomfortable and has a few more risks. No one likes to have a probe passed into his or her esophagus.

During this examination, two or three electrodes, placed on the chest, continuously monitor the rhythm of the heart. An IV, usually placed into a vein in the arm or wrist area and attached to tubing, allows fluid and medications to be given directly into the bloodstream for immediate action. An *oximeter*—a small device placed on the finger—monitors the oxygen level in the body. Supplemental oxygen is usually given to keep the blood oxygen level high during the test. The gag reflex is usually suppressed with a spray numbing the back of the throat. Medication is used to relax the patient, but he or she may feel the tube as it is passed through the throat. The flexible tube is gently passed through the mouth and into the esophagus while the patient lies on his or her left side. Images are obtained. The exam usually lasts about 15 to 20 minutes, depending on the information needed.

There are more risks for the TEE than a regular echocardiogram. The main risk comes from the IV medications given: an adverse reaction or side effect could occur. Also, any time an IV is started, there could be a very small risk of bleeding. When the probe is passed into the esophagus, there is a minimal chance of damage to the teeth or the back of the throat. To minimize these risks, close monitoring is required. The test is usually performed in a hospital because of the mentioned monitoring devices and possible risks, but the patient usually goes home the same day. The patient might have a sore throat after the procedure. The numbness should leave the throat before eating is resumed.

In preparation, one must have an empty stomach because there is a risk of vomiting during the test. If on a daily medication, I have my patients take their medication at least two hours before the procedure. Because of the risks involved, the provider gives a very detailed explanation to the patient. The provider will request permission by way of a consent form to be signed by the patient, stating that he or she has received an explanation and understands the test and the risks involved. As you can see, the risks are not too great, but they are present. Every precaution to minimize and understand risks should be taken before the exam.

Heart Catheterization (Coronary Angiography)

Cardiac catheterization is a test in which a small plastic tube called a *catheter* is positioned at various locations within the heart. The information acquired includes visualization of the coronary arteries and any blockages that might be present, the strength of the heart, and measurements of pressure within the heart. The procedure lasts from 30 to 60 minutes.

This test gives the cardiologist a great deal of information and often provides definitive answers regarding cardiovascular system abnormalities. For instance, if a stress test is abnormal, heart catheterization can verify the results of the stress test and gauge the severity of the problem. The procedure determines the nature of blockages in the arteries, indicating the best treatment to be recommended. The information regarding the strength of the heart and the pressures within the chambers is also very useful.

In preparation for the procedure, the risk and benefits are explained—just like I am doing now—and the patient is asked to sign a consent form. Blood is drawn to make sure blood counts are good, the kidney is functioning well, and there are no clotting abnormalities. An EKG and a chest X-ray are usually performed to provide baseline data. If diabetes, kidney disease, hypertension, or other adverse medical conditions are present, your provider may give specific instructions. You will be advised concerning which medications to take before the test. A written medical history is completed before the test to give your information to those who may need it.

Ideally, the stomach needs to be empty before the procedure. If the procedure is scheduled as an outpatient, I ask the patient not to eat anything after midnight. He or she can have sips of water to take their regular medications. Sometimes an adjustment on diabetic medications needs to be made. The patient must have someone drive him or her home after the procedure.

The actual procedure is performed in the hospital or a special outpatient center. If not already in the hospital, when the patient arrives, an IV is started in a holding area. The patient should go to the bathroom before entering the catheterization suite. Sometimes, a urinary catheter is inserted into the bladder in females. If the patient is to be given relaxing medications, it usually will be done at this point. The chart is reviewed to make sure all preliminary preparation has been completed.

The catheterization suite is the room where the procedure is done. The patient will be positioned on a table that is surrounded by an X-ray camera, which will take the pictures. The camera will move to various locations during the procedure. There will be several monitors, usually on the left side of the patient. This enables the cardiologist to visualize the heart, observe pressures within the cardiovascular system, and monitor the heart rhythm. The patient might see a control room where technicians assist with the procedure.

After the patient is placed on the table, electrodes are positioned on the chest to monitor the heart rhythm. The area over the right and left groin will be cleaned and shaved. A drape will be placed over the entire body. This will help keep the procedure clean (sterile). The technician will hook up the needed equipment. At this point, if the patient has not been given a medication by mouth to relax him or her, it will be administered by IV. The patient will be awake during the catheterization, as the medical team will need to communicate with him or her.

Injecting a medication called Xylocaine with a small needle will numb the area over the entry site, usually the right groin. Other entry sites are sometimes needed, depending on the circumstances. The numbing feels like a large bee sting. The cardiologist will give numbing medication over the entire area. At this point the patient should start feeling relaxed and should feel no significant discomfort. The cardiologist then places a small device called a *sheath* into an artery. The sheath is used to carefully pass catheters (long, thin, plastic tubes) into or near the heart. This will allow data to be gathered. The patient does not feel the passing of the catheters. The cardiologist is able to see where the catheters are going by looking at a monitor.

Special contrast material (dye) is injected into the coronary arteries and X-ray pictures are taken. The contrast material allows the arteries of the heart to be seen by the X-ray. These pictures are then recorded for future review. Numerous pictures from different angles will be taken. The strength of the heart is measured by placing contrast material into the left ventricle, and pictures are obtained as the heart pumps. This may cause a very warm sensation, or "hot flash," as the contrast agent is pumped throughout the body. If needed, pressures in various parts of the cardiovascular system are measured.

After the diagnostic procedure is finished, the patient will go to a recovery area. If no emergent treatment is needed, the sheath will be removed. Some cardiologists hold direct pressure over the entry site for about 20 minutes, until any bleeding stops. Other cardiologists use a special device, which is inserted into the artery, sealing the hole created by the sheath. In this case, direct pressure is not needed. The patient will then have to remain fairly still, lying on his or her back, for several hours after the procedure. If the patient needs to use the bathroom, a urinal will be provided.

While in a supine position (lying on the back), the patient will be monitored closely for bleeding. If there are no complications, the patient may eat, but must still continue to lie fairly flat. After a certain amount of time determined by the cardiologist, the patient will be able to move around and go home, pending the results of the test. After going home, the patient should be careful to limit physical activities. The cardiologist will give specific discharge instructions.

A heart *catheterization* is termed an *invasive procedure* because the catheter is considered to be "invading" the body. There are definitely more risks than in the previous tests described in this chapter. The risks include, but are not limited to, the following:

- Adverse reaction to the medication given for relaxation
- Bleeding at the entry site
- Damage to the blood vessels from the sheath and catheters
- Damage to the kidney from the contrast material
- Heart attack
- Stroke
- An adverse reaction to the contrast material
- Abnormal heart rhythms

There's even a small risk of death, and the risk of a serious complication is also very small. I would not recommend this test unless the benefits of knowing what is causing the symptoms outweigh the risks.

Electrophysiologic Testing (EP Testing)

I need to briefly mention a sophisticated form of testing the electrical system. EP testing allows the cardiologist to determine if the electrical system of the heart is malfunctioning. The specific causes of a malfunction can be identified. This test might determine whether the electrical system is firing too slow, too fast, or is irregular.

A specialized cardiologist, called an electrophysiologist, performs this test in a laboratory very much like a catheterization suite. The procedure is similar to the heart catheterization previously described. However, in this procedure, specialized catheters are placed at various positions in the heart where information on the electrical system is obtained. Sheaths are placed in a vein or in an artery in the groin area. The catheters are passed through the sheaths into exact locations in the heart.

This test is recommended for any of the following symptoms:

- When an individual has had a cardiac collapse relating to the electrical system
- If previous testing has demonstrated certain types of dangerous rhythm patterns not managed with medications
- If further information relating to the electrical system is needed
- When a heart has been declared very weak

In some situations, the electrophysiologist can use energy to destroy certain electrical cells of the heart that are causing the abnormal rhythms. This is called an ablation. At other times, small devices that monitor the heart and restore normal rhythms—should an abnormality develop—are implanted. These devices are called automatic internal cardiac defibrillators.

The test is longer than a regular catheterization, but the preparation is similar. However, in addition to the risks mentioned for a regular heart catheterization, there is also the increased risk of causing a dangerous heart rhythm. Again, this test would not be done if the benefits of testing did not outweigh the risks.

More Sophisticated Tests

In the past few years, a number of more sophisticated tests to evaluate the heart have been developed. These tests are growing in use and availability.

The following is a list of these noninvasive tests, along with a brief description of each test.

1. Multisliced Computerized Tomography (CT scan of the heart). This test uses X-rays and computerized processing to make pictures of the heart and other blood vessels in the body. There are new advanced scanners, called *Ultra Fast CT Scanners,* that can visualize the coronary arteries. This may lead to early detection of coronary artery disease. The benefits are currently being evaluated. There are minimal risks. This test may be able to replace the need for heart catheterization in many instances.

2. Magnetic Resonance Imaging (MRI). This type of advanced test uses a magnetic field to make images, rather than using X-rays. Most MRIs use a moving platform in a circular tunnel and are quite noisy. Some people feel claustrophobic in these machines. New circular open MRIs have been developed. The MRI gives detailed information on the heart structures. This test is used infrequently.

3. Carotid Ultrasound. This common test uses sound wave energy to provide information regarding the large arteries of the neck—specifically looking for blockages in these arteries. Ultrasound can also look at the large artery in the abdomen—the aorta—as well as the arteries of the legs, to evaluate for abnormalities.

4. Echocardiogram With Contrast Agents. Sometimes special agents are given through an IV while an echocardiogram is being performed. Contrast agents are used when a regular echocardiogram does not show the heart structures well. These agents enable the cardiologist to better visualize the heart structures. The preparation is the same as that for a regular echocardiogram. There is a small risk of an adverse reaction to the contrast agent.

5. Positron-Emission Tomography. This is sometimes called a *PET scan,* and provides detailed information about blood flow to the heart. Radioactive material is given through an IV, and a sequence of images is made and recorded. The machine rotates around the body to capture many images. The patient will be in a supine position (on the back) in a device that looks like a large doughnut. PET scanning is very expensive and its availability is limited. This test is rarely used in the evaluation of the heart.

Myths About Cardiac Testing

A negative stress test means I cannot have a heart attack. This is not true. A stress test may be positive if significant blockages are present in the coronary arteries. However, there is a chance that a significant blockage (or blockages) will not be picked up by a stress test. Currently, there is not a test that can predict who will have a heart attack. Risk factors help us identify persons who are more likely to have a heart attack. Maybe someday we will have such a test.

If an EKG is normal, my heart is fine. This may or may not be true. You could be having a heart attack with a normal EKG.

Ask Your Health-care Provider

This concludes an overview of the most common—but not all—diagnostic tests of the cardiovascular system. Keep in mind that if you have specific questions regarding any test ordered, you should ask your health-care provider.

Treatment

Once a diagnosis is made, treatment is individualized. The treatment plan should keep in mind a person's needs and preferences. There are many "right" treatments, but it is beyond the scope of this appendix to list every treatment for every condition. I will mention some helpful, general principles.

Remember, knowledge is power. The more you know, the more you will be able to participate in your own care. We'll discuss the more common medical responses, beginning with acute treatment. *Acute treatment* is what must be done immediately.

Coronary Artery Disease (CAD)

Blockage in the arteries supplying the heart with blood is termed *coronary artery disease* (CAD) or *coronary arteriosclerosis*. We've discussed symptoms and tests that represent and confirm CAD. CAD is the most common problem leading to a malfunction in the cardiovascular system. I'm going to explain CAD in a little more detail because a better understanding will help you learn about the treatment.

Every minute, a person dies from CAD. It's the leading cause of death in every community in America. This is also a growing worldwide problem. The problem develops because the coronary arteries become narrowed or blocked completely. When this occurs, blood with oxygen (nourishment) cannot reach the muscle. Typically, symptoms follow.

What causes the arteries to be narrowed? Your body carries fats called *lipids* in the blood. Lipids can gradually build up inside the blood vessels. These buildups can become hardened, or *calcified*. Other elements become involved as well, making the blockages bigger and bigger. Blood has a hard time passing through the arteries and cannot reach its destination. When the heart muscle does not receive enough blood, symptoms develop. We discussed these symptoms in Appendix 1.

Before we go on, I want to make a few points. The blockages in the arteries of the heart can also be occurring elsewhere in the body, including the arteries supplying the brain, legs, and other vital organs.

Sometimes a blockage—also called *plaque*—may become unstable. If this plaque, which you can think of as an artery "pimple," pops, there could be big problems, even if there is just a 30 to 40 percent narrowing in the artery.

When the "pimple" pops (ruptures), the body sees this as an injury. If you had a cut on your arm, other cells would be recruited to fight the damage. Inside the arteries, cells are recruited to help fight the damage when a plaque ruptures. These cells mean to do well, but as they congregate around the rupture, they can clog up the artery, leading to a heart attack.

Mr. Adams is a 40-year-old who had never had a medical problem in his life. One morning while getting ready for his job at the electric company, he developed excruciating chest pain. Testing revealed that a 30 percent plaque obstruction inside a coronary artery had ruptured, causing a heart attack.

Unfortunately, there are no diagnostic tests to predict which plaques will rupture. If we had this test, we could predict all heart attacks. When Mr. Adams' plaque ruptured, the recruited damage-fighting cells formed a clot that resulted in a loss of blood flow in the artery. Severe pain resulted.

Mr. Adams' problem was diagnosed quickly and treatment was initiated. The cornerstone in the treatment of *acute* CAD is to first restore blood flow to the heart, and then help prevent further problems related to the lack of blood flow from developing. *Chronic* treatment involves trying to halt or even reverse the disease process. This is called *regression* and is usually accomplished through diet and other lifestyle changes.

If blood flow is not restored quickly by opening the blocked artery, a heart attack will occur. This could lead to many serious problems. Because of the lack of blood flow to the heart, the electrical system could be damaged causing dangerous fast or slow heart rhythms to develop. When these rhythms occur, the heart might be beating so fast or slow that it is unable to pump blood throughout the body. In a heart attack, the heart muscle itself does not pump well because of an insufficient supply of oxygenated blood. Without oxygenated blood supplied by the heart, organs of the body cannot function.

The heart valves controlling the direction of blood flow depend on muscles that may be damaged during a heart attack. Blood flow might move in the wrong direction because the valve is not working properly. This is another major acute problem.

During a heart attack, it is even possible that a dead heart muscle may break open or rupture. This event is usually fatal. As you can see, getting immediate treatment could save your life.

If you think you're having a heart attack, sit down, call 911, and leave the phone off the hook so your call can be traced if you pass out. Take a blood-thinning aspirin if possible. Try your best to relax. Do not drive yourself to the hospital. If a ambulance does not take you to the hospital, let everyone know when you arrive that you think you are having a heart attack.

The acute treatment for a heart attack will focus on restoring blood flow to the part of the heart not getting blood, as well as treating the resulting problems previously mentioned if they occur. Aspirin and oxygen will be given. Emergent catheterization is often performed. This will help in deciding whether the artery needs to be opened by a procedure called *angioplasty*. This might be the first treatment option initiated, pending the situation and availability. Sometimes clot-busting medications (*thrombolytics*) will be given through the IV to help open the artery. Other medications to help the heart and prevent blood clots will be given, based on the patient's condition.

Angioplasty (PTCA) uses the technique of heart catheterization. A catheter is inserted through an access point in an artery (usually in the groin) and is passed to the origin of the coronary arteries. Pictures of the arteries are obtained. In addition, a guiding catheter is passed to the blocked coronary artery.

Next, a second catheter with a balloon near the tip of the catheter is threaded through the guiding catheter. The balloon is inflated to squish the blockage against the artery wall and restore blood flow. The balloon may be inflated several times. A small metal device called a *stent* is usually placed (deployed) in the artery to help keep it open. A drug-coated stent is usually placed to help keep the vessel patent (open) long-term. These devices, which look like a spring and are made of stainless steel, are designed to hold the artery open and help prevent further narrowing of the vessel, or restenosis.

The procedure has more risks than a heart catheterization. The cardiologist performing the procedure will explain the risks. Drug-coated stents, along with medications to help prevent clotting, have greatly decreased the amount of restenosis and have enhanced the treatment of acute myocardial infarction. During and after the procedure, strong medications are administered to help prevent clotting and keep the blood thin.

In addition to angioplasty and stents, there are other procedures currently used to open arteries. *Atherectomy* is a process by which a device removes the fatty plaque in the artery. This is sometimes called a "rotor-rooter" procedure. The plaque is scraped away using a special catheter. The plaque is either pulled out of the body or ground into very small particles and carried away by the bloodstream. Lasers are used infrequently to help open the coronary arteries.

Angioplasty and stenting are the most common procedures used to open arteries. However, these procedures do not remove the chance of a heart attack; they allow more blood flow through the coronary artery, which helps the heart get more oxygen so that serious problems previously mentioned may be averted.

Bypass surgery (more on this later) is sometimes needed if angioplasty is not successful, or if severe complications result from the heart attack. If the heart has an abnormally fast rhythm, the heart will need to be shocked (defibrillated) to restore a normal rhythm. If, during the heart attack, the heart is going abnormally slowly, a device called a *pacemaker* will help speed up the heart. Medication is also given to help stabilize the abnormal rhythms.

After the initial event, the patient will be admitted to the hospital for several days for an uncomplicated heart attack. If there are complications, the hospital stay will be longer. The medical team will begin medications to restore optimal heart function. Preventive measures will be initiated. Finally, the activity level will gradually be increased and cardiac rehabilitation will begin.

Only about one fourth of the people who could benefit from a rehabilitation program actually participate in such treatment. Rehab programs help all patients with heart disease and are a very important part of the treatment plan. The program serves to educate concerning the cardiac condition—to counsel, support, and teach preventive measures. In addition, the patient's physical activity will be gradually increased under a monitored situation. I cannot overemphasize the importance of a rehab program in an acute treatment plan.

Diagnostic testing might reveal that one or more of an individual's arteries are partially blocked and that a heart attack is looming in the future. Specific treatment will be individualized. For instance, if blockages are not too severe, medications will be given to diminish the demands of the heart, along with aspirin and a cholesterol-lowering medication. If medications, preventive measures, and lifestyle changes are ineffective in controlling symptoms, a more invasive form of treatment may be recommended. In situations with severe blockages in the arteries, an angioplasty or bypass surgery is recommended.

Sometimes medical therapy cannot control symptoms. If there are severe blockages in multiple coronary arteries, or the main branch of the coronary system is blocked, a bypass surgery is recommended. It's important to note that some arteries are so severely diseased or so small that neither bypass surgery nor angioplasty would be beneficial. Heart catheterization gives this information to your health-care provider.

In the past 25 years, coronary artery bypass surgery (CABS) has become a common treatment for diseased arteries.

Coronary Artery Bypass Surgery

CABS involves taking an artery from the chest wall, or sections of veins from the legs, and attaching them to coronary arteries below the severe blockages, giving more blood flow to the heart. The transplanted bit of artery or vein is termed a *graft*. In some situations, arteries may be taken from the arm.

An artery tends to have fewer problems over time than veins from the leg, which are accustomed to lower pressures. Arteries have stronger walls, too. This new connection brings a new blood supply to the heart. Removal of the conduit (graft) will not usually significantly affect blood flow in an individual's body.

A specialized surgeon, a cardiothoracic surgeon, performs the operation. A general anesthetic will be given to put the patient to sleep. For the surgery, different techniques are available. Traditionally, the chest is opened through the breastbone to reach the heart. The patient is placed on a special heart-lung machine when the heart is not beating. The machine takes over for the heart, which is stopped during the surgery.

The surgeon then places the grafts. If a vein is used, it's attached with very small stitches (sutures) to the aorta, the large artery leaving the heart, which is full of oxygenated blood. The vein is then attached to the coronary artery below the severe blockage. If the artery in the chest (called a mammary artery) is used, it is attached directly to the coronary artery below the blockage. This artery is already full of oxygenated blood.

When all the grafts are completed, the patient is removed from the heart-lung machine and the heart is restarted. After this, the breastbone will be put back together with stainless steel wires.

Recovery takes place in an intensive care unit. After the patient is discharged from the hospital, postoperation recovery is usually six to eight weeks, but varies from person to person.

If bypass surgery is needed to treat CAD, the surgical team will supply detailed information regarding the risks and recovery. Today, new techniques using smaller incisions are being used. In certain situations, surgeons may opt to sew the bypasses into a beating heart, and the bypass machine is not needed. In this type of surgery, the recovery period is usually shortened.

Before ending this section, there's a need to reemphasize that in the acute treatment of CAD, the ultimate problem is severe blockages that prevent adequate blood flow in the artery. After the acute treatment is completed, these blockages must be addressed by preventive measures, which may help the blockages become smaller (regression) and more stable. Whether the arteries can be acutely treated successfully by angioplasty/stents or bypass surgery can be a difficult decision, with more than one "right" treatment available.

All the specific medications used for treatment of acute CAD have not been covered. It is important for you to know, in general, that medications for CAD (1) lower and stabilize cholesterol levels, (2) lower the risk of clot formation, (3) increase blood flow to the heart, and (4) decrease the workload of the heart. The workload can be decreased by medications that slow the heart, lower blood pressure, and dilate the arteries.

Chronic Coronary Artery Disease

Because much of coronary artery disease is acquired, I would like to focus on its treatment. Simply put, we develop CAD largely because of daily decisions made throughout a lifetime. Once we have it, we must look at our lifestyle and evaluate the choices we've made and are making.

Coronary artery disease—blockages in the arteries supplying blood to the heart—is the most common manifestation of a disease in the cardiovascular system. Much could be written about the chronic treatment, but I'll keep it short, and hopefully sweet.

We must lower cholesterol with good nutrition sometimes used in concert with medications. When I say "good nutrition," I mean ideally a plant-based diet. We must also include daily exercise, maintain optimal body weight, keep blood pressure low, stay away from cigarettes and secondhand smoke, limit stress in our lives, and laugh as much as is humanly possible. That's right. Laughter is good for the heart!

It's hard to admit that we give a disease to ourselves. While genetics do play a role, it all comes down to the choices we make in taking care of those genes. Diet is a very personal subject. Our Westernized diet—high in fats and refined food—contributes greatly to CAD. What's high in fat? Meat, eggs, cheese, and milk are major players in the development of CAD.

Also, the Western diet is high in sodium. What contains sodium? It's not so much the table salt that we sprinkle on for taste. It's the packaged, processed, canned foods that contain extremely high amounts of sodium and other chemicals that our body was not created to handle.

In parts of the world where a plant-based diet predominates, CAD is greatly reduced—sometimes nonexistent. As the world has become "Westernized," the disease rates in those same areas have skyrocketed. It only makes sense that the cornerstone of the treatment of chronic CAD must involve optimal nutrition.

Exercise does so many wonderful things for the body that it should definitely be considered as a treatment. There are even times when exercise proves to be more effective than medications. Daily exercise helps to lower the blood pressure, increases "good" cholesterol, lowers the "bad" cholesterol, diminishes stress levels, helps prevent and treat diabetes, and keeps the weight down. And if that weren't enough, exercise also keeps the inside lining of the blood vessels healthy. The list could go on and on. I think you get the point that exercise is vital in treating chronic coronary artery disease.

Treating stress is also very important in the management of chronic coronary artery disease. Chronic stress damages the body in many aspects. It can cause development of bad coping mechanisms such as smoking, drinking alcohol, using recreational drugs, and overeating. Stress hinders rest, raises blood pressure, and causes headaches and muscle pains throughout the body. Stress also increases the chance of experiencing a heart attack. Believe me, treating stress is crucial to the successful treatment of chronic coronary artery disease.

There are many other ways to treat coronary disease, including getting appropriate rest and maintaining proper fluid consumption. However, do not forget the big three—nutrition, exercise, and stress. Combating this disease demands a change in our chemical environment, which can be accomplished by the above methods. But how do we change a lifetime of bad habits and poor choices?

The power to do that can't be found in us. It can only be found in God. He gives us the power to make changes one at a time as we learn to depend on Him daily. This divine power is essential in not only the treatment of coronary disease, but also the achievement of our life goals. Studies have confirmed that patients with an active spiritual life do better in their personal lives.

As we gain the power to make changes, we begin to feel better. This enables more and more positive changes to take place. Our chemical makeup will shift as we eat better, exercise, and deal with stress. The disease becomes stabilized, and even—incredibly—regresses. Yes, this disease can be reversed! The treatment of chronic coronary disease requires discipline, hard work, and power from God.

As patients make these changes, they tell me they feel better than they have ever felt in their lives. They wouldn't go back to their previous habits for any reason.

Remember, our habits and the way we live contribute greatly to the problem. Even though we can place a stent in an artery or bypass around blocked areas, we must examine the larger picture and deal with the long-term aspects of the problem. If this is not done, the problem will recur. Let me repeat that. IF THIS IS NOT DONE, THE PROBLEM WILL RECUR.

Now that we have discussed the treatment for chronic blockages, the most common problem in the cardiovascular system, let's move on to other treatments of the cardiovascular system.

Malfunction of the Electrical System

When the electrical system malfunctions, the heart goes too slowly, too quickly, or irregularly. The heart does not generate adequate pressure to pump blood to the body.

The malfunction is diagnosed as described previously. For abnormally slow heart rhythms, if no outside sources are causing the problem (for example, medications), a pacemaker is recommended. A *pacemaker* is a small metal device consisting of a battery, electric circuits, a computer-like sensor, and leads. The battery is placed under the skin, usually in the left upper chest area near the collarbone. The leads are thin wires attached to the pacemaker. They are directed into the right side of the heart. At the tip of each lead are electrodes that sense the heart's activities and send electrical impulses if needed. Pacemaker placement is done under local anesthetic (numbing medicine and a medication to relax).

Pacemakers help the heart beat sequentially by sending electrical charges, causing the muscle to contract when needed. The pacemaker contains sensors, which can monitor the heart's activity. Based on these sensors, the pacemaker may or may not send electrical impulses. These devices are now very small, about the size of a matchbox, and can last approximately six to eight years, depending on the situation. The function of the pacemaker is evaluated over the phone monthly and visits to the cardiologist at six-month intervals.

An external control system is used to make adjustments. I can't think of a more important device than a pacemaker to extend the life of a patient. People with pacemakers can participate in sports and live active lives. A pacemaker card is carried at all times in the rare case of a malfunction.

In other electrical abnormalities, the electrical impulses speed through the heart too *fast*. A variety of treatments are available. At times, avoiding stimulants such as caffeine, cigarettes, or alcohol can treat rapid rhythms and palpitations. Any type of stress to the body including pain, emotions, or illness can cause the body's own natural signals to make the heart skip and beat faster.

Many medications are available for the treatment of rapid heart rhythms. The type of fast heart rhythm detected and the patient's overall medical status determine treatment. The health-care provider should discuss the pros and cons of these medications with you.

An abnormally fast rhythm can be treated by *cardioversion*—a jolt of electricity from an outside source used to reset the heart. During this process the patient is mildly sedated—unless under an emergency situation. Two paddles or electrode pads are applied to the front of the chest or the back. An electrical current is passed through the heart. Hopefully, the heart will reset to a normal rhythm. Sometimes the chest feels sore afterward.

There are occasions when groups of cells in the upper part of the heart can produce a fast, abnormal heart rhythm. This can be thought of as a "short circuit" in the system. Electrophysiologic testing can identify the cause of these fast rhythms. A specialized cardiologist, called an *electrophysiologist*, can localize where these abnormal rhythms are coming from. These areas can be destroyed permanently with the use of sound waves in a process termed *catheter ablation*.

In some individuals, abnormally fast heart rhythms begin in the bottom part of the heart. These are often life-threatening. Devices called *Implantable Defibrillators* can be placed to help correct this problem. These are similar to a pacemaker, but are slightly larger and made of titanium. They sense the dangerous rhythms and fire electrical impulses to terminate the abnormal rhythm. The impulse, or "shocks," can be uncomfortable. Special instructions are given to patients with defibrillators. The defibrillator has various programs to deal with abnormal rhythms. Ex-Vice President Cheney recently had a defibrillator implanted while in office.

Heart Failure

When the heart cannot pump adequately to meet the body's needs, heart failure is said to occur. There can be many different causes of heart failure. The muscle may be weak because of blockages in the arteries; the heart may be unable to relax; the electrical system may malfunction; toxins such as alcohol, chemotherapy, and radiation may damage the muscle; or the valves may function inadequately. There are a host of other causes including, but not limited to, infections, thyroid disease, medications, and sometimes inherited disease.

Treatment focuses on correcting the underlying cause, if possible. In addition, many medications are available to help a weak heart. Some of these medications help by blocking the hormones a failing heart initiates, because a high level of these hormones can damage the heart further. In addition, lifestyle changes are recommended, including monitoring fluid intake and avoiding salt. Too much fluid or salt can overload the heart. Usually your provider will recommend an exercise program. Recently, special pacemaking devices can be used to help certain weak hearts. These are called biventricular pacemakers.

If these measures are unsuccessful in controlling symptoms, some individuals may be eligible for heart transplantation. This would be a last resort, as donors are scarce. Before a transplant is considered, strict health criteria are followed, including the exclusion of other serious health problems.

Valvular Malfunction

If a heart valve malfunctions and symptoms develop, the valve needs to be replaced or repaired. The timing of surgery is crucial to long-term success. A valve should not be replaced or repaired too soon because there are risks involved in open-heart surgery. Conversely, if one waits too long, the heart may be weakened, leading to a more difficult surgery and recovery. A cardiologist will advise you in regards to timing. Often medications can be used to treat milder valvular problems.

It's important to determine whether a valve can be repaired instead of being replaced. If surgery is needed, a cardiovascular surgeon, along with a cardiologist, will determine the best replacement valve for you. There are numerous heart valves available, including both mechanical valves and tissue valves. Each valve has its pros and cons that should be discussed before surgery.

This appendix does not mention treatments for every malfunction of the heart, but a general overview has been given. There's constantly new research for the treatment of heart disease.

Lately, there's even been research and evaluation into a new artificial heart. A left ventricular assist device is now available, which can help a weak heart pump blood. Some surgeons are removing dead heart muscle to improve heart function. Researchers are injecting growth factors into the heart to grow new blood vessels. Some researchers are using lasers to make small holes in the heart to assist it in obtaining more blood. New medications are being developed for the treatment of heart disease. In the future, we'll possibly be hearing more about gene therapy as a method of treatment.

Myths About Treatment of Cardiovascular Disease

Once I've had bypass surgery, I cannot have a heart attack. This is false. Your risk is still present, but because of increased flow from the grafts, the heart attack tends to be smaller.

THE HEART OF HEALTH: AVOIDING DECEPTION

Medications can prevent a heart attack. Certain medications lower the risk, but do not prevent it all together.

Medications
Following is a list of the types of medications used, along with the effect on the heart.

MEDICATION CLASSES USED TO TREAT HEART DISEASE

ACE Inhibitors (angiotensin converting enzyme inhibitors)	Block the production of natural substances that cause blood vessels to narrow, thus lowering blood pressure. Also used to treat heart failure; help the heart to heal after heart attacks.
Alpha blockers	Relax the muscle around arteries, lowering blood pressure.
Angiotensin II (receptor blockers)	Lowers blood pressure by blocking receptors that are used to constrict blood vessels; may help patients with weak hearts.
Antiarrhythmics	These medications help control abnormal heart rhythms.
Aspirin	Inhibits blood clotting by interacting with platelet function. Used to treat CAD.

Beta blockers	Block receptors that result in a slowing heart rate. Used for hypertension, CAD, and CHF (conjestive heart failure).
Blood thinners	Work in different ways. Help prevent blood clots from forming. Used in many situations.
Calcium channel blockers	Relax blood vessels, and some can slow heart rates. Used in hypertension, CAD, and in some rhythm problems.
Cholesterol-lowering medications— statins, fibric acid, niacin, and binders	Decrease cholesterol levels. Used to treat CAD. Some of these medications have been shown to reduce the risk of heart attack.
Digitalis	Increases contractions of the heart; can slow heart rate. Used in CHF and some arrhythmias.
Diuretics	Lower blood volume by increasing the amount of sodium and water removed through the kidneys. Can also cause loss of potassium. Used for hypertension and CHF.
Fibrinolytic (clot dissolver)	Breaks blood clots used in acute myocardial infarction (heart attacks). Most useful when given within a few hours of a heart attack.

Inotropes	Increase the pumping ability of the heart. Used in CHF.
Nitrates	Help the coronary arteries to dilate, and lower pressures in the heart. Useful in CAD and CHF.
Platelet receptor inhibitors	Block the ability of platelets to stick together and form clots. Used in CAD. Help prevent clot formation around stents.

Medication Pearls

If your doctor prescribes medication, it's important for you to have a working understanding of the following:

- Know why you are taking each medication and what the medication looks like.
- Understand the directions for taking each medication.
- Get prescriptions refilled at least a week before you anticipate running out.
- Know which medications, if any, have caused you problems.
- Keep medication in original container in a cool place.
- Don't take medication in the dark.
- Don't stop taking a medication without talking to your doctor first.
- If you have surgery, dental work, or emergency treatment, tell your provider which medications you are taking.
- Don't double up on a medication without advice.
- Never share your medications with others.
- Get all prescriptions filled at one pharmacy; they will have a complete record.